The Hole

by

Andy Frazier

A short novel adapted from a screenplay of the same name by the same author, completed in 2016.

GW00391357

Version 1.2 - Removed markup lines

Printed 02/03/2020

Andy Frazier

For livestock farmers, everywhere.

The Hole

September 2001 - Great Orton Airfield, Cumbria

Watching the great machine at work, the Brigadier wiped his brow, his eyes squinting in the low evening sun. It had been a long task, much longer than he or anyone could have possibly imagined. Much harder too, and he had seen a lot of hardships during his forty plus years in the forces.

As the vast bulldozer shuddered past, its tracks squeaking from over-use, the vibration of the ground underneath him took his mind briefly to what was below: thousands upon thousands of carcasses. How long before they all decayed? How long would it be before they were forgotten? How long before the horror faded?

He suspected it would be decades, if not centuries.

Mid February 2001 - Newcastle, England

It is a chilly winter's morning as Dennis drives carefully along the streets of Ponteland, past all the posh houses where all the footballers live. They weren't up yet. He suspected most of them rarely saw dawn unless they were just coming home from nights out on the 'toon'. Talk about overpaid? The wages these guys were on would settle the national debt in a fortnight? A grey cat darts across the road, tearing him from his thoughts as he touches the brakes and the wheels lock up on the ice. 'Steady,' he mutters to himself.

Shortly he swings the van into the airport, gathering speed now he is on roads that had been gritted to clear the ice. Ignoring the signs for the main entrance and car-parks, he pulls down a side lane and eventually slows as he reaches a checkpoint, winding down the window.

'Morning Bob, bit of a chilly one, eh?'

'You're not wrong, Dennis, brass monkeys today, that's for sure.' Bob presses a button and the barrier slowly creaks up to allow his passing. 'Mind how you go, eh?'

Dennis just raises a hand and moves forward, heading round towards the backdoor to the airport, a place where few ventured, especially not this time of day. Reversing the van into a loading bay, he jumps out, climbs the short ladder and grips the first of the large grey bins that are standing outside some bigger roller-shuttered doors. Inside the building, the kitchen staff are already at work, preparing meals for the busy day ahead and he can hear chatter as steam seeps through the door, creating an eerie mist. At first the metal container refuses to budge, its wheels frozen. Dennis gives them a kick and tries again. This time the bin rumbles along as he shoves it with both gloved hands towards his vehicle. Once he has opened the back doors, he manoeuvres the bin onto a ramp and into the back, securing it with a strap. He repeats this with two more similar ones, ensuring the lids are firmly shut, and heads back into the dark, nodding to Bob the security guard as he passes through the barrier once more. Turning off the A696 he takes the side road towards Heddon-on-the-Wall, a route he does three times a week. There are a few cars on the road, commuters using the lane as a rat-run, off to work in Newcastle or further afield, but generally it is quiet for the couple of miles until he reaches the A69, one of the country's main arteries.

A minute later the driver arrives at his destination, an entrance at the pig farm marked by black letters carved in stone. The van's headlights illuminate a row of long wooden buildings, each one with a metal grain storage hopper at the end. The animals had been sleeping but the sound of his engine, coupled with the motion sensor lights coming on soon boot them into life. As he pulls into the yard, amid a cacophony of squealing, the smell of the pigs catches his nostrils, while he pushes open the van door and reverses back into a loading bay.

As he wheels the last bin into place, he braves lifting the lid to peer inside, and then recoils, wishing he hadn't.

'Bloody hell, that's minging,' he says out loud to nobody in particular. His voice is lost amongst the sound of hungry creatures, as he heads back into the van and leaves in a hurry. It wasn't a job Dennis enjoyed.

An hour later, two workmen wheel the bins along to the pig sheds, pouring the mixture of offal and food waste into large troughs.

'There you are, me luvvlies,' one says, as the pigs tuck into their breakfast. 'All good and fresh for ya.'

23rd February 2001

'That was the latest single from those oh-so-spicy Spice Girls,' a smooth DJ speaks from the lorry's radio speaker. 'But don't go far now, as we have a rock-and-roll classic coming up, right after the news.'

Neville Lambert rolls down the window, pulls a cigarette from a half-used pack and lights it, his bare tattooed arm resting on the window ledge. A glare of bright sun peeps over a hillside, occasionally dazzling his eyes as he squints for better vision, while the artic lorry rumbles along a narrow lane, bordered by mountains on either side speckled with sheep.

The news reporter starts his morning's recital: 'Reports are just coming in about a suspected outbreak of foot and mouth disease in South West England. No official details have yet been released but it is thought to be in sheep on a farm in Devon.'

Neville doesn't give the matter much thought as he runs his hand through his spiky hair and pulls up alongside a farm driveway, the brakes squealing as the wheels slow to an abrupt halt. Finding reverse gear, he effortlessly guides the 40-foot, three deck livestock trailer backwards into the narrow drive and down a tight muddy farm track towards some buildings.

'Morning Mr. Donald.' Neville unlocks the ramps, lowering the tailboard. Eric Donald just nods, clad in oilskins as he leans on a railing, a ruddy complexion beneath his flat cap catching the light from the morning sun. He is flanked by two eager but obedient collies. Once the gates are opened the first of a flock of ewe lambs immediately starts to trot down the lorry's ramp towards the farmyard, Neville counting them with two fingers as they go. Eric is counting too, he knows that, although the old man is showing no physical signs of it. Neville suspects the dogs are probably counting as well, just to be sure!

Another five minutes, after all the decks have been lowered on electric motors, the last of the bunch trot down into the fresh air.

'242. That right?' says the driver. The old man just nods his head, looking towards his new flock. 'Some decent lambs, Mr. Donald.' Nev continues, 'Should grow into some bonny ewes.'

'Bloody well aught to be at that price,' Eric speaks for the first time, his voice gruff and steeped in a hardened monotone Galloway accent.

Nev had been to this farm a few times, delivering and collecting livestock, and he can rarely remember the old man saying more than a few sentences during that time. Most of these hill farmers were men of few words. Nev wonders at the limited conversations Eric and his wife would have over dinner, as he brushes the sawdust from the ramps, folding aluminum gates across each other and eventually raising the ramp. 'Right you are then, Mr. Donald, that's me.' The two men nod to each other again as Neville climbs back into the cab and starts the engine.

A couple of miles along the road, he picks up his

mobile phone and hits an autodial button.

'Hi Helen, can you hear me?' he looks at the screen. 'How's she doing?'

Nev shakes the phone and mutters, 'Bastard things, never work when you need them.' Narrowly missing an oncoming car, he pulls the truck into a layby and tries again. 'That better? Can you hear me now? How's that ewe doing?'

Nev listens to his wife's reply before speaking again. 'I am supposed to be back in Carlisle this afternoon, but I think I'll just come by home first and take a look. What?' Shakes his head. 'Don't be saft woman, nobody's going to know. I'll just tell them I got lost...'

Within half an hour Nev swings the lorry into a smallholding known as Newhouse Farm, near the village of Auldgirth, in Dumfriesshire, turning in a circle to face the way he came in, and then reversing it straight near the fence. He glances towards the house to see his wife watching him arrive from the kitchen window, before climbing from the cab and entering a small paddock via a newly erected gate. As he scans the field he sees what he is looking for and slowly makes his way towards a rotund ewe lying on the grass, straining. When he judges that he is near enough, Nev pounces on her, catching her by the back leg as she springs to her feet. Eventually he grapples the ewe to the ground again, glancing his head off a stone. The sheep is pushing out a prolapsed womb which he puts his hand on. 'Steady girl. C'mon now. I'm not going to hurt you.'

Nev hears his wife calling from by the field gate. 'Are you alright, Love. You need a hand?'

'Of course I need a bloody hand!' he replies through gritted teeth, as he is struggles to hold the ewe down and push the womb back in. The first drops of rain from a storm splatter on his forehead. 'Do I have to do bloody everything round here?'

Helen crosses the field towards them wearing a heavy coat, wellingtons and woollen hat. Silently she takes hold of the ewe's head releasing Nev's hand so he can attend to the job.

'Will she be OK?' Helen's voice is calm, with a mild Scottish lilt.

'If she keeps doing it, she's going to need a stitch in there to hold it in.'

'Isn't that a job for the vet?'

'Vet? I can't afford a bloody vet.' Nev's voice goes up an octave, ' You're a nurse, can't you do it?'

She puffs out her cheeks. 'I suppose I could try.'

Shortly Nev lets go of the ewe which stands up and wanders off. Together they watch her before Helen goes to put her arm around her husband. He shrugs it off.

'Have they been fed?' he asks, curtly.

'Yes, of course, at daylight, as always.' Helen avoids adding a hint of sarcasm to the sentence, knowing how stressed Nev is already and suspecting his hot-headed reaction. Helen fed the sheep every morning, before taking the kids to school, despite her battle with morning sickness now she was seven months pregnant. Hers had been a life of hard work around sheep for as long as she could remember. It was him who was the novice, not that she ever raised that subject. She knew he worked hard too and was trying to make better of himself.

Half an hour later the pair of them are back at the table in the kitchen of their modest bungalow, Nev nursing a cup of warm tea while spoon feeding Sophie with one hand. The two-year-old grabs at the spoon, as though she was starving, and then smears the runny mixture around her mouth, grinning.

Helen is at the stove with her back to him. 'Did you hear the radio? A suspected outbreak of foot and mouth?'

'Aye. I heard it. But it's down south somewhere. Won't affect us up here.'

'I hope not.' She turned to face him, concerned. 'But it's quite scary, isn't it? I mean, that stuff spreads so fast.'

Nev sniffs, watching the child. 'It's nothing to worry about, trust me. Probably just a few lame yows and an over cautious vet. Nothing's been confirmed. We've got enough to care about just now. You know what she cost don't you. That yow. Eight hundred quid, that's what.'

'Yes, I know. I know what they all cost.' Helen turned back to the stove, to avoid eye-contact for the oncoming conflict.

'What's that supposed to mean?'

'Nothing! I just mean that I know they were expensive ewes and we have to do the best we can with them.' She turns to him. 'She'll be OK, won't she? It's just a prolapse. As long as we keep checking? It's still four weeks till lambing.'

Nev calms a little and sighs. 'Well I hope you're right. If she loses those twins that's a quarter of the flock gone.'

Helen has him back under control again, but he is still on a knife edge. 'It's not quarter of the flock, don't exaggerate. Do you want my Dad to come and look at her?'

When Nev bangs his fist on the table it takes her by surprise.

'No, I don't want your bloody Dad to look at her. I don't need him here lecturing me on how we should be keeping Blackies instead of this new-fangled Beltex breed.'

'He said he'd help. We only need to ask. '

'I don't need help.'

'He has a lifetime's experience and he…'

Nev pushes the chair back getting to his feet and eyeballing Helen aggressively. 'I said I don't need bloody help! OK?' he shouts, before storming out of the door, slamming it behind him. Sophie starts to cry.

For the next few hours Helen busies herself in the house. She is used to Nev's outbursts, but he never got violent, not with her anyway. In fact, she prides herself that she is the calming influence to his more audacious streak, the yin to his yang, and it somehow seemed to work. Sure, there have been times when he has gone over the top and she has walked out but once the air had cleared there was always a shared blame somewhere in the middle-ground. Generally it was about money, or lack of it, but still they had achieved far more than anyone expected of them, which was mostly down to him. And he loved her, she was in no doubt of that. Since the day they had met, Nev only had eyes for her, she was convinced of it.

By the time evening comes around, Nev arrives back into the yard in his pick-up, checking the ewes before he comes into the house, washes his hands and sits down for his dinner. With the kids in bed they talk in a civilized manner about nothing in particular, him doing the dishes while she tucks the kids up. A move into the sitting room, feet up, TV on, as couples did the world over. Nine o'clock, time to see what was going on in the world of other people.

Andrew Bird shuffles his papers on TV before staring straight into the camera, and from there into people's homes, his city suit immaculate as always. The music dies away giving him his cue to speak. He doesn't look cheerful, but then the news wasn't exactly a comedy show. Especially not tonight.

'Yesterday's suspected case of foot and mouth disease has been confirmed by the Ministry of Agriculture this evening. In all 17 sheep were found to be affected on a farm near Wadebridge in Devon. The sheep had been transported by lorry from Longtown market on Tuesday. Other animals that have travelled from the same source are to be inspected today. All infected animals will be slaughtered immediately.'

The screen cuts to a flock of sheep innocently standing in a field, followed by a shot of animals in a market that could have been anywhere. In the sitting room at Newhouse Farm, Neville Lambert drops his cup to the table, pulling his hands up through his spiky hair.

'Fuck!' he stands to his feet. 'Fuck, fuck, fuck!'

Helen appears at the door. 'Nev, for god's sake. The children can hear you!'

He doesn't even acknowledge her. Opening a pack of cigarettes and lighting one nervously. 'Shit. What have I done?'

'Neville. What? What is it? What's up?'

'The lorry, that's what's up. The fucking lorry. I brought it here.' By now he is at the window, looking into the darkness beyond.

'I know you did. I saw it.' She replies, still calm. 'What of it?

'Those lambs. That load. Fuck!'

Still not quite grasping the problem, she raises her voice. 'Nev, calm down. What about that load?'

'I picked them up in Longtown!'

Helen stares at him, and using her mother's sternest voice says, 'Neville, sit down and tell me what this is about?' Before he could speak she was collecting the cup, now lying on its side, and mopping the table.

Nev sits back down, staring unblinkingly towards the ceiling. His voice is shaky. 'The news just said that a load of sheep from Longtown Mart had taken foot and mouth to Devon. I just picked up a load from the same market and brought them to Dumfries.'

As Helen heads to the kitchen, she whips around, the information sinking in as he continues. 'I just brought foot and fucking mouth to Dumfries!

Taking a deep breath, she tries to rescue some calm, eventually putting her arms around him, perching on the side of the chair. 'It's not your fault, Nev. It's your job. You were only doing your job. Doing what you were told.'

A tear welled in Nev's eye. 'I didn't just bring it to Dumfries, I brought it here, to our home!'

'How? What do you mean?'

'Don't you understand? That stuff spreads. You said it yourself. That stuff, that invisible fucking cancerous stuff. It spreads on anything it touches.'

For his wife, the penny was starting to drop. 'The lorry?' she almost whispers it. 'You think it can spread on the lorry?'

'Not just the lorry, Helen. On me. I handled 300 sheep and then came home and handled one of my own. One of my own special yows.'

Nev stands to his feet, making for the door. Outside it is dark and raining as he runs across the yard, shouting. He has a torch in his hands. As he reaches the gate the sheep are spooked and run.

'I killed them.' His shouts penetrate the night. 'My pride and joy. The first decent animals I have ever owned, and I fucking killed them.' One sheep trips as he sees it in the spotlight, limping a couple of steps. He drops to his knees and screams. 'Fuck!'

The word echoes around the hillsides.

The Hole

24th February 2001

Some hours after Helen has gone to work, Neville sits at the kitchen table with a mug of tea. On the side surface sits a small portable TV that has previously been in the bedroom and barely used. The sound is turned down as Neville speaks into the phone.

'Yes, Mr. Armstrong, I understand. How long do you think it will remain closed? A week? Really. Well, is there any other driving jobs I can do? I have to feed my family, ya na.'

The voice on the other end is no more reassuring as Nev swallows the words before replying. 'OK, well if anything comes up, I'll take it. Please. Right, Mr. Armstrong. Yes, I hope so too. Bye.'

Putting down the receiver, he lights another cigarette and crunches up the empty packet. The phone rings again and he grabs it.

'Yes! Oh, it's you. Yes, I haven't forgotten. What? Oh for Christ's sake, Helen, yes!' He stands restlessly, waiting for a chance to continue. 'You want the good news or the bad? Good news is the prolapse has stayed in and that I can't see any lesions on the sheep's mouths. Everything looks OK but how can I tell? I checked the internet but there's all sorts of shit on the MAFF site. Haven't heard any more about Eric Donald yet, we have to sit and wait. No, Helen, that is the good news. The bad news is Armstrongs just laid off all of their drivers until further notice, so I am out of a job.

No real surprise there, I suppose.' Barely hearing her response, he continues. 'No idea. At least the rest of the week, maybe more. They are still paying a basic, but with no mileage bonus, it's going to be tight. Carlisle Mart is still operating so might see if they will take me back on as a drover for a few days. Hang on…'

Nev picks up the remote and turns up the sound on the TV before speaking back into the phone. 'OK, pick up Sophie at 2 and George at 5, got it. Ok bye. What? Yes, I will, bye.'

A pretty female newsreader is centre screen above a huge red banner with the words FOOT AND MOUTH CRISIS. Doing her best to remain expressionless, she reads from the autocue into the camera.

'Four more cases are now confirmed, two in Devon and two in Cumbria. It is thought that animals taken to Longtown market, possibly pigs, have spread the disease. MAFF officials say that any animals that have come into contact with the disease will be more or less guaranteed to have contracted it. Due to the nature of the modern way of farming, animals are continually transported across the country in lorries like these, often in cramped conditions. Jeffrey Barnett from the Farm Animal Welfare Council spoke to us earlier:'

The screen cuts to man in a snow-white jumper with grey beard in clean wellington boots. 'Outbreaks like this are inevitable until someone stops these appalling conditions in which animals have to live...'

Nev has had enough already and erupts. 'That's it, have a go at the farmers. Any excuse to have a crack, you bearded twat. Stick the knife in, why don't you? I don't see you complain when lamb is cheaper than coal. But then you probably don't eat meat anyway do you. I hope you choke on your tofu, arsehole!'

He stands up and goes to the sink, washing up a cup and putting the kettle back on with his back to the TV. The programme has cut back to the newsreader. 'Other news, Prime Minister, Tony Blair, visited Newmarket in Suffolk this morning. With only six weeks to go until the General Election, polls show that the Labour Party is 12% ahead of its nearest rival.'

Nev scoffs at the TV without turning around. 'And you needn't bother either, you poncy pillock. Since when did you care about anyone except yourself? Haven't seen you out there helping us farmers lately. Or anyone else north of Watford.'

Tony Blair is being interviewed, smiling smugly. 'Well, it isn't exactly a crisis is it? Just a few isolated cases. Our team at MAFF, which was recently moved into new facilities by the Labour government, have the whole thing well under control. And furthermore, our leading vets are expert in such matters. Yes, a few animals will be culled but the countryside will still function as normal.'

Nev shouts at the screen. 'Function!? Is that all we can do, bloody function? The countryside feeds you townies, pal. You need reminding of that.' The phone rings again and he turns the TV sound off.

'Yes. Really?' He opens a new pack of cigarettes. 'What all of them? The whole fucking load? Jesus, Ron. Is that really necessary? Poor Eric, they were some bonny beasts. Oh well, I suppose he will get some sort of compensation? He said they were too dear anyroad.

Alright.' His pal continues on the other end for a few more seconds before Nev replies. 'What? Disinfectant. I've probably got some Dettol, somewhere. What do you mean, sold out? Are you telling me Carrs have sold out of disinfectant in one morning? Really? OK, I will get Helen to pick some up in Carlisle. Thanks for the call, Ron. Yes mate, and you.'

The day passes slowly as Nev ponders the situation, punctuated only by him going out to collect the kids from school and nursery. By evening he doesn't really relish the thought of going out to his darts match at the Old Station, but Helen persuades him he should, to take his mind off things.

The pub is busy by the time he throws his darts to finish the first game with a score of 64.

'Good arrows, mate,' says his opponent, begrudgingly. Nev takes his handshake and makes his way past a few others before sitting back at the table in front of a half full glass.

Next to him his pal swigs his own beer. 'Still got your eye in then, partner?'

'Aye well. A few of these helps,' Nev replies

Ron's eyes narrow a fraction. 'As long as it's just a few, mate.'

Nev drains the pint and moves to a fresh one. 'If ever there's been a time to drown the sorrows, it must be now, eh?'

'How's things back home? How's Helen?' Ron asks above the noise of the pub.

'Ah, ya na. She's getting bigger, hormonal, uglier!' He

grins as Ron elbows him in the ribs.

'Nev, your missus is the prettiest thing this side of the Forth Bridge, and you know it. And she works like a donkey, nursin and bringing up kids while you are out truckin your way round the country. Far too good for the likes of a rough-neck like you!'

Nev gives him a hard glance and then smiles. 'Aye, ya right I suppose. Ganna be hard times just now though, Ron. I dismissed this disease to start with but looks like it's got the wind up its tail now.'

Ron runs his hand over his near bald head, 'The yows still OK?'

'Aye. Far as I can tell. Hey! Nobody is to know I brought that truck home yesterday, OK? Those trigger-happy bastards are just as likely to turn up at my door else.'

Ron shakes his head. 'Mum's the word from me mate. I just hope that stuff didn't come with you, for all our sakes. Did you get the disinfectant in place?'

'Aye. I spread some straw across the gateway like they said and dowsed it. Put some at the field gate too. You think it will do any good? Nobody seems to know how this stuff is spreading. Some say on the wheels, others on the wind. S'like putting up a net to hold out the tide.'

Ron nods thoughtfully and then his eyes lighten a little. 'They're paying out. You heard that? Government has announced they will compensate full price. Sending out valuers onto all farms at risk.' He lets out a laugh. 'Trust those buggers at Carlisle Mart to keep their jobs going even when the Mart is closed.'

Nev looks him in the eye as if to check it isn't a wind up. 'Closed? I didn't hear that. I was thinking of getting some work there.'

Ron continues, picking up his glass again. 'Aye. Shutting the whole country down tomorrow afternoon. Nae movements of any animals without a licence. Announcement just now.'

A portly man in his forties sits down at the table beside them, joining into their conversation. 'What's that, Ron, shutting the country down? Says who?'

'Well, not all the roads, obviously, Gerry. Just all stock movements.' Ron tries to make light of it, seeing the solemn look at Gerry's face. 'Shouldn't affect your business mate, you'll be sound where you are. It's just that this foot and mouth is spreading and the government are panicking.'

Nev shifts in his seat, raising his voice. 'Government? Don't get me started on that one. Those arseholes in London wouldn't know a cockerel from a cockroach. Sending out a few beardies in white overalls from MAFF to review the situation. The need to act, Ron. Never mind paying out, they need to snuff it out. This thing is like a hedge fire, once it gets hold all their hot air will just fan the flames.'

The red-faced man who Nev had beaten at darts, turns up with a fresh pint. 'There you go, pal.'

'Cheers, John.' Nev nods. 'Beat you fair and square back there.'

John accepts the thanks. 'How you getting on with those fancy French sheep of yours?'

Nev looks surprised. 'They're not French, they're

from Belgium, not that you would know the difference, having never been south of the Solway.'

The man squares up to him. 'French, German, whatever, they're all the same, those foreigners. Probably them that sent this disease over, just for a laugh. You know they'll be closing all the roads next because of you farmers, putting me out of a job an 'a.'

Nev let go of his pint, tightening his fist until Ron put a hand on his arm. 'Don't let em get to you. You've done and seen more in your young years that that old bugger will have ever read about. He's just concerned about the local community, they all are.'

Nev was apprehensive. 'Did I do the right thing, Ron? Buying the yows I mean. Spending all our savings. You can tell me I'm wrong, Ron. You're a proper farmer, mate. It's in your blood to know about these things. Look at me, just a chancin bastard from a Carlisle council estate.'

Ron smiles. 'Oh, you kin me. I'm just a cattle man. Sheep all looks the same to me.' He laughs out loud at his own teasing. 'Although those ones of yours do look more like hippos than the sheep these folks are used to.'

'They certainly got some meat on them.' Nev laughs too. 'I just saw them at that sale and thought they were right, somehow. You know, something new for a new millennium. A fresh start. Helen's old man nearly fell off his crook when he saw them. Says we'll never get the lambs out without a tractor puller!'

Ron drains his beer. 'Aye, he may be right. My Belgian cows are the same, have to drag the buggers out. But if they're worth calving, they're worth keeping, that's what I say.'

'Well, they've done you no harm, have they. What was it, six grand for a bull last year?'

Ron just raised an eye in recognition of the fact that his herd of Belgian Blues was possibly one of the best in the North. 'Here's hoping we get to hang on to them.'

26th February 2001

Helen pulls the car into a space in the school car-park, checking her hair in the mirror before getting out. Since she had turned 30 last year, she was aware that her girlish good looks had started to fade, and she can see bags under her eyes just like her mother's, especially since the pregnancy with her third child progressed. She steps out of the car just as Alison Priestly is passing, immaculate as always in her pearls and cashmere. Helen straightens her nurse's uniform.

'Hi Ali,' she says. 'How's things?'

Another woman has already come over to join them as Alison speaks. 'Helen, you're a farmer, tell me this isn't serious? This, this cow thing?'

The other mother joins in. 'Yes. It won't affect us, will it? And are you sure we can't catch it?

By now, as in primary school playgrounds throughout the land, another mother has come to join the gossip, laughing. 'My Charlie is convinced he has it already. Tried to get the day off school this morning!'

'Well, I would be lying if I said it wasn't serious.' Helen tells them, trying not to alarm. 'To our livelihoods, that is. Well to ours anyway. My husband is quite worried as it seems to be spreading. He believes we should all take as many precautions as possible to stop the spread.'

It was Alison who took the remark most gravely.

'Do you think we should get some disinfectant set up at the gates to the Garden Centre? Gerry was considering it.'

'Can't do any harm, can it. You must get quite a few folks in there who have been near livestock.'

'Not as many as we used too.' Alison sighs. 'Sales are definitely down over the last week or so.'

Charlie's mother takes the chance to get her concerns heard. 'Do you think they will close the school? I don't know what I would do if our two had to stay home. I just don't have the money for childcare these days.'

Another mother concurs. 'Me neither.'

As the first of the children start coming out of the main doors Helen turns away from the others, seeing her son George. She walks him to the car, taking his bag. 'Have a nice day, George?'

George climbs into the passenger's seat and looks down at his satchel. 'No!'

'No? What's up?'

George doesn't look up, as he speaks quietly. 'Daniel says sheep are stupid. He says they are stupid and dirty. And that they spread diseases.'

Helen hadn't anticipated this and takes her time to answer. 'Just ignore them, George. They don't understand what's going on. They are all a bit worried, that's all.'

'They don't, do they, Mum.' His eyes are misty. 'Sheep don't spread diseases, do they?'

Meanwhile, at the other end of the country, the same question was being discussed in a bit more detail. Number One, Whitehall, London, is and had been for many years, home to The Farmers Club. Meetings had been held here for centuries on a range of topics amidst agriculture's corridors of power. Its high-ceilinged rooms brag about the opulence of days gone by and an industry that was extremely profitable and dominant in society. Large ornate curtains frame massive windows looking out to the city while golden guilt framed portraits hang systematically around its wood panelled walls, depicting men of power through the ages. Currently the men of power include Minister of Agriculture, Ralph Green, and his head vet at the ministry, Professor David Prince, amongst its elite, the latter of whom is sitting at his desk awaiting the former. As he is served coffee by a man in white uniform, the door opens and Green enters.

'David, good to see you,' comes a somewhat false greeting.

'Minister,' says David, subserviently.

The minister puts down his briefcase on the leather topped table and sits. Whist a coffee is also poured for him he takes out a single-sheet memo and reads it. 'So, reading between the lines here, everything is under control?' His gaze stays on the paper.

It is all David can do to stop himself from sighing out loud. 'I am not sure where you see that, Sir. We have some of the cases isolated but there is no sign of the spread abating.'

Green glances up for a second. 'Let's look on the bright side, David. Only a few isolated cases. Nothing to get too alarmed about, eh?'

'With the greatest respect, Sir, although we don't have all the facts, I think we need to err on the side of caution.' Prince can barely contain his frustration. 'This is a particularly virulent strain, not like the ones we have seen before. It seems to be some sort of mutation and spreads in different ways to the strains we have been studying.'

'So, you are saying it is spreading?'

'Er, yes, that is what I just said.'

'So, we don't have it under control.'

'No. Not yet.'

'I see.' Green strokes his chin. 'And what are _we_ doing about that?'

Prince goes for broke. 'I need more help, Sir. More resource. A team.'

Predictably the minister rises to the bait. 'You have a bloody team, David. We set it up last year. Nice new offices, shiny laboratories, computers, bums on seats. Isn't that a team?'

'We can't control it from our seats, Sir. This needs men out in the field. And vets. Quite a lot of them.'

'Oh, don't talk such bullshit. There are plenty of vets out there in the...' Green gestures to the window, 'countryside, all looking for a bit of extra work. Just hire a few, give em a couple of rifles and go and knock out these infected creatures. God dammit, we just fought a war, David. If we can beat those damn Arabs, I am sure we won't let a few sheep cause too many problems?

Silence impregnates the air for just a little too long for comfort for either man. Prince takes a breath before delivering the lines he knows will shake the tree. 'It's not that simple, Sir. We can't just shoot the animals until we have a valuation done, and then MAFF authority in each case. That is taking a few days. And then we have to dispose of them.'

Predictably, Green's face reddens. He pulls his large frame up from the chair. 'In each case. We only have a dozen bloody cases, man. Just do it.'

'48, Sir. As of an hour ago. 48 cases.'

'Well act quicker then? Speed up the process.'

Prince shifts uneasily. 'The problem isn't our end, Sir. It is at yours. Your people have to sign the cheques, not mine.'

Green sits down, again, thinking. 'So, how much more resource do you need to make this thing go away. You do know we are coming up to election time? Few hundred thou? A million, maybe.'

'I can't actually say, Sir. But we certainly need assurance that if we take on more staff, they will get paid for. And - pardon my expression - a kick up the arse for your finance department.'

Immediately Green replies, 'The PM won't like it.'

'He'll like it even less if we have to shut down the whole country.'

Ralph Green quietens for a second, his eyes narrowing to slits as he eyeballs his subordinate. The next sentence he pronounces slowly and intensely. 'Did you just threaten me, Professor?'

Letting the words hang in the air, Prince doesn't back down as was expected of him. 'By all means tell the PM we are doing all we can, but...'

'No fucking 'buts', Professor Prince. End this thing, or I will find someone who will.'

The outburst takes Prince by surprise but still he keeps his cool. 'There is another way, Minister. We both know that.'

'Which is?'

'Vaccination.'

Green rises from his chair again, the anger rising with him. 'What? Spend millions vaccinating every cow and sheep in the land?'

'It's a valid option.'

'An option which would mean economic suicide.'

'In the short term, perhaps,' Prince knows he has the man rattled now, as he throws another verbal punch. 'But it would save a lot of animal's lives.' Already he was anticipating the answer, despite the script that had been prepared for the media, but it was worth a shot, if only to see the man squirm a little.

'This has been discussed and ruled out. If we vaccinate, we admit to the rest of Europe that we have an inherent problem with foot and mouth disease and nobody this side of the fucking moon will want to buy our meat. Not now, not ever!'

Prince waits with his answer, although he knows it won't be heard. 'We would get over it, Minister. Eventually.'

Green slams his fist down so hard on the desk that the chandelier rattles overhead.

'No, no and no. It won't happen. Just get what you need and end this thing now. Do your job man, or so help me I will hang you out to dry. Understood?'

1st March 2001

Darkness was hanging in the air as though reluctant to shed light onto such a gloomy morning as three unmarked white vans follow in convoy down a narrow tarmac road. As they near the buildings, the road is barred with a gate displaying a sign saying FOOT AND MOUTH DISEASE - ENTRY PROHIBITED. Chief veterinary officer, David Lawson, opens the door of the first vehicle and gets out, pulling on white overalls and wellingtons. Half a dozen other men do the same. Nobody speaks for a full minute until David takes authority over the crew, just about making out the shadowy figures in the dim light.

'Ok men, we have been through this already. Any of you new to it, stick with someone who has been here before. Where's Reed?'

Jim Reed, an athletic man in his early 40s, red hair concealed under a woollen hat, steps out from behind another van, zipping up his suit.

'Over here boss.'

Lawson issues instructions. 'Take two men and get them armed. I'll go and see what we have.' He pulls a clipboard from the van and checks it, before opening the gate and entering the farmyard. The silhouette of a man approaches them through the darkness. 'Ronald McCall? Are you the proprietor of this High Church Farm?'

Ron pulls his flat cap back from his head, looking directly at him. 'Aye, that's me.'

'David Lawson, Ministry of Agriculture, we have a requisition from the government...' Lawson recites a script he has used a number of times before.

Ron cuts him off. 'Aye. I know who you are and why you're here. Just come in and get on with it. Cows are all in the byre.'

'Can you sign here please?' Lawson holds out a clip-board.

While Ron signs the papers four more men in white overalls come through the gate, two carrying rifles. One of them is Nev. As they pass him, Nev touches him on the arm.

'Sorry, mate.'

Ron doesn't answer, just looks away, his eyes welling up. The four men wander towards a barn, which is lit by a floodlight highlighting the steam rising from the beasts inside. Nev glances over to the house to see the face of a woman at the window, tears streaming down her cheeks.

Lawson's voice rings out through the mist. 'Clean shots, lads. Let's have no fuss. It's not a job that anyone wants to do, so let's get it over with.'

Turning his back on them, Ron walks towards the house, going inside and closing the door. The kitchen blind closes. Out in the yard the men go about their business in a routine fashion.

Nev assesses the situation, finding all the cows in a large stone open fronted building. The rifle he has been given is one he has seen many before, which used to be standard army issue 303. Modern guns had outdated this one now, but it was still efficient for this purpose. He loads one bullet into the chamber as two other men alongside him fill up their magazines. Resting on the gate, he takes a look through the telescopic sight, breathing very shallow. He takes aim on a large cow in one corner of the shed. Her yellow ear-tag displays the words Belgian Blue, along with some numbers. Underneath that, written in indelible marker-pen is the word Bluebell. She looks at the man with his gun in a knowing way and Nev swallows, tightening his finger on the trigger. Above the noise around him, he can hear his own heart beating in double-time, adrenaline rising without warning.

Nev closes his eyes.

Now he sees a range of mountains glowing in an early morning light below which are miles upon miles of desert. The whole place appears to be deserted but his tele-sight tells him differently. Amongst the darker caves on the hillside over a mile away, the crosshairs meet on a man sitting cross-legged with an AK47 rifle in his hand. Beneath the towel around his head, Nev sees the face of a young teenager, possibly no more than 14 years old. The youthfulness of the man looks eager to please, doing a job he was born to do, as his fearless eyes scan the nearby land, checking, watching, ready to report or defend his master. Nev's heart is still pumping double-time. He too has a job to do. Orders to follow. One squeeze is all it takes. The man drops sideways. Job done.

Around him, shots rattle in the darkness. Nev opens his eyes, taking his bead on the cow once more. A single shot pierces the centre of the animal's skull.

His voice is barely whisper. 'Sorry, mate!' Putting down the rifle he rubs his eyes and hands the rifle to one of the other guys. 'Take over, mate, will ya. I'll be back in a minute.'

Crossing the yard to the house he glances back at the byre where 20 cows are lying together, some still moving. A lot of them are bleeding, although shots are still being fired, some into the carcasses. He catches sight of Bluebell, lying still as though asleep and stops to take a breath. David Lawson catches up with him.

'Everything alright, lad?'

Nev turns to him, his eyes bloodshot. 'He loved that beast, ya na. She meant the world to him.'

The man returned his stare. 'She was sick, Neville. It had to be done.'

Screwing up his eyes, Nev lets out the emotion that has built up inside him. 'There was nothing fucking wrong with her! You're a vet for Christ's sake, how can you do this? How can you let this happen? This is murder! There was nothing wrong with her. Nothing wrong with any of them. Only thing wrong here is your fucking rules. Your rules that say she might be infected because some farm down the road had the disease.'

Lawson stayed calm. 'You didn't have to do this job son. You volunteered.'

'I volunteered to help. This isn't help. This isn't helping anyone. That guy is my mate. What help is this to him. We're not the solution, we're part of the fucking problem.'

'He'll get compensation.' The vet eyed the ground. 'That's how it works.'

'Compensation? How can you compensate for years of breeding? How can you compensate for hours of love and kindness? How can any government compensate from killing anything, anyone? All they needed was a vaccine, mate. Not a fucking war.'

'Neville, I don't really think that is your concern. You are just doing a job here. The rules aren't made by us, we just carry them out.'

Nev has calmed down a little. 'You said so, yourself, Mr. Lawson. You admitted that a vaccine could stop this disease in its tracks. Didn't you say that?'

'I am not the law, Neville. I just abide by it. I suggest you do the same if you want to keep on working for me.'

The two men face-off, rain drizzling down, until eventually Nev breaks the stare. 'Ron is my pal. I only came on this one today to make sure they did it right. Those cowboys you have working for you are a disgrace. Couldn't hit a barn wall from inside the barn. At least Ron's best cow got a quick death.' He starts to walk away then turns to continue. 'Now if you don't mind, I will just go and tell him it's all over, Mr. Lawson. All over for him now, at least. Maybe he will take his cheque, and take his family on holiday to the Caribbean, away from all this madness, while the rest of us swim through the shite.' After a few more yards he stops again, pointing toward the cow byre. 'Except it isn't over yet, is it. Not till they get rid of all that lot.'

Sometimes the skin feels dirty, long after it has been cleaned. That's what Nev felt like that evening, as he scrubs away at his with a hard brush in the steamy shower. Taking twice as long has he normally would, eventually he steps out, dries and dresses then joins Helen and the children at the kitchen table.

Helen pretends not to notice how red raw his bare arms are when he sits down, but she knows him well enough to know he had a really upsetting day. 'Poor Ron. He has worked so hard for that farm. What will he do now?'

Nev looks towards the windows, fixing his gaze on nothing in particular. 'I told him to get away on holiday but you know what he's like. Married to that place, married to those cows. It will be like losing a wife!'

'Steady.' She splutters. 'He can buy more cows!'

'You know what I mean. I suppose time will heal. And that cheque will help a little. Seems they valued up quite well. 1200 apiece for the cross-breds, he wouldn't get that in a market. And four grand for Bluebell.' He continues to stare into space for a while, recalling the blue cow he shot. 'I took her out, with one shot. Did I say?'

Helen holds his hand across the table.

'You did the right thing, love. From what you say, those cowboys wouldn't....' She drops the subject, turning to her son. 'Anyway, it's over now. Eat your dinner, it's getting cold. George got a gold star today, didn't you George?

The boy looks excited. 'Yes, for drawing a picture of a sheep.'

Nev isn't listening. 'But it isn't, is it? It isn't over yet, because they have to shift those carcasses. Killing the animals is the easy part. You know what they're doing, don't you? They're burning them, right on the side of the yard. Piling them up and setting fire to the lot right where Ron and his family can watch. What fun that must be for the kids?'

'They haven't got much choice, have they. What else can they do?' Helen stiffens slightly.

'Can you imagine the smell? The stench of burning flesh, once smelled, never ever forgotten.' Nev stands up and looks out of the window. 'Believe me. Never forgotten! And that still isn't the end of it, is it? Because that smoke. That toxic smoke spirals up into the air and then drifts on the wind. Then it drops again, into the valleys, carrying its germs.'

'I'm pretty sure they said it can't spread via the smoke, Nev. Didn't they say that?'

'Oh aye, they said that. They said a lot of things, didn't they. But what if they're wrong. What if they just make that shit up, just to keep us quiet. What then when my ewes get lined up in the crosshairs? What bloody then, eh?'

'We should be safe up here, shouldn't we?' Helen isn't convinced by her own statement.

'Safe? Safe? There's me getting exposed to that stuff every day, just so I can put food on the table. Then bringing it home with me.'

'But you wash, don't you?' she replied. 'I've seen you scrubbing, so hard it makes you bleed, Nev. And the disinfectant? That stuff stinks so bad, the whole place reeks of it. I can't see any germ surviving the amount you use. And you don't bring your clothes home.'

'Well, one thing's for sure, I'm not going near those yows myself,' he sniffs. 'Not while I am doing this job, no matter how many times I have washed. It's up to you now, Helen. You're my eyes and ears.'

Helen gets up to go to the sink. 'They're still a couple of weeks off lambing yet, Nev. Hopefully all this will be over by then, won't it? Everything back to normal?'

'I wish. Can't see them stopping this mess just now, especially these local lads. I think half of them want it to spread. Keeps them in a job, doesn't it? And not all farmers are like me either. Some of these hill boys have been struggling for years. Wouldn't say no to a nice pay-out and a holiday.'

'You're saying some farmers want to get the disease? I don't believe that.' She spins around, shocked.

Nev is calm again now, being reflective. 'Well think about it. Struggling to make a living? Can't even take stock to mart to pay some bills. Going out in all weathers to feed stock that might get killed next week anyway. Chance of a fat cheque from the government, doubling the value of your cows?'

'You're not saying Ron did that, are you?'

'Nah, Ron wouldn't do a thing like that. Anyway, there was no evidence of the disease in his cows, not that I could see. It seems they culled him because the farm next door had it. A contiguous cull. That's how it works.'

'Well, at least we don't have any neighbours.' Helen comes across and puts her arm around him.

But Nev isn't finished. 'Ah, but we do, don't we? We

have this whole hillside as a neighbour.'

She recoils again. 'You're not saying they would cull the entire hill. Those blackie ewes have been up there for generations!

'I wouldn't put it past them! Then what? If they go, so do we?'

'But the hill ewes never come near us, Nev. They rarely even venture on to this side of the mountain?'

'Won't matter, will it. They are our neighbours, no fences to stop them coming this side of the hill if they wanted to. We'd be next in line.' Nev lets out a laugh. 'One thing's for sure, those cowboys wouldn't be up to that job. Getting near those yows would take a military sniper.'

Car headlights swing round in the yard outside. Nev stands and goes to the window. 'Who the hell's that, at this time of night?' He wipes the glass. 'Bloody hell. That's all I need.'

Out in the yard, Tam Campbell steps down from his pick-up, pulling his sheep crook from the seat beside him and zipping up his oil-skinned jacket. He isn't in a rush, as he glances around the yard and then over to the house. Tam was never a man to rush and at top side of 60, he wasn't going to start now.

Helen meets him at the door. 'Dad. What are you doing here?'

'Och, just passing,' his accent is broader than hers, the smoother edges worn rough by too much time spent on foggy hills. 'Thought I'd drop by, see how you're coping.' He nods to Nev. 'Neville.'

'We're coping just fine thanks, Tam. Everything under control here. Not needing any help, just now, ta.' His tone is curt enough to be noticed but calm enough not to appear rude.

'Good to hear it. Ewes all OK?'

'All fine, thank you.' He turns towards the television.

Helen helps her father off with his coat. 'Can I get you a drink, Dad?'

The old man removes his wellingtons on the step in the porch and leans his sheep crook by the door post. A sure sign he was certainly staying for a few minutes at least. 'Och, well. Just a quick dram. I'm won't stay long mind,' he winks at Helen, 'or your Mum will think I am in the pub!'

'She knows you too well.' His daughter smiles.

Tam takes a seat at the table. 'Baby all fine, Helen? Taking it easy?'

'Aye. Fine. Had a scan a few weeks back. All in order and on track for a couple of months time.' She blushes slightly. 'Still working just now but I'll give up in a few weeks, once this problem dies down a bit.'

Tam nods slowly. 'I heard about your job, Neville. That's unfortunate, son. Might be a good few weeks before this all gets back to normal.'

Helen comes to his rescue. 'Nev's been doing some work for the Ministry, haven't you Nev?' She pours two whiskies for the men and sits down.

Nev lights a cigarette and sighs. 'Aye. Been out with the cowboy gang for a few days. But it's not for me. That crowd couldn't run a piss-up in a distillery.' He swills the whisky around in the glass and sniffs it.

'No? I thought they could use your skills? Just the sort of lad they need.'

'Trust me, Tam. They need more than me. A lot fucking more.' Nev drains the whisky and stands up, pulling on a jacket. 'Just check the yows and it's bed for me.'

Tam stands, draining his glass. 'Mind if I hae a look?'

'Aye, if you wants.' Nev mumbles his reluctant agreement.

Picking up his coat and crook Tam follows him out into the yard. The pair of them look over the gate and the ewe has prolapsed again.

'Bollocks! I thought she'd stopped that.' Nev climbs the gate and goes towards her, opening a small pen and managing to get her inside. He inspects the red bulge hanging from her back end while Tam stands back, outside the gate, just leaning on his crook in the drizzle, saying nothing, letting his son-in-law deal with it.

Eventually, Nev looks across to him. 'Go on, then. You know you want to. Give me a hand, or some advice, or whatever you came here to do.'

Tam still doesn't move, just leans on his stick. 'You're doing fine, son. All I want to do is see you and the lass succeed, that's all.' He then remains silent, watching Nev push the prolapse back in, and then tying it with string. Once he has it secured, Nev comes back out to the gate and Tam resumes. 'You might not believe this, lad. But I admire you for taking a chance. For having a go. For standing up for yersel tae get what you want.' The older man turns and walks back towards the house and then stops. 'That's nae my breed o choice, but I'm old school. You know that. Too much o the hills in me tae be putting sheep intae sheds. But I'm sure they hae rights to a place in this world. And so do you, laddie. So do you.'

2nd March 2001

For more than two generations, farmers throughout the country have relied on a few common basics to get them through their day and two of the most essential of have been the Land-rover and baler twine! At 63 years old, Henry Wilson would have been reaching retiring age, were he in any other profession. After all, he had two sons, one married and living in an old worker's cottage on the farm. The other had left the trade, but not gone too far, choosing a career as a farm rep for a local feed merchant.

Henry had taken tenancy of the farm when he was the boy's age, and, with the help of the bank, managed to buy it from the landlord for a sum far less than it was valued today. In fact, his bank manager had recently told him what the farm was actually worth, and Henry had nearly fallen off his comfy chair in the man's comfy office as he sat through an annual meeting with the bank. However, what the manager had also said was that Henry wasn't making ends meet, and that his cows were failing to turn a profit for the second year running, if he took into account feed costs, fertiliser, repairs to building and machinery etc. Couple this with running two households, things were getting harder, year on year. And now, as if a hard winter hadn't kicked him enough, there was a country in crisis, a restriction order on moving any animals, and no chance of selling anything to pay the sixty-day old bills that were mounting up his sideboard.

'Come on! Come on!' he shouts over a ramshackle gate that may well have been nearly as old of himself. Untying the frayed string that held it closed, he lifts a bag of feed from the old Land-rover, which was certainly older than his sons, and calls the cows again. Soon they arrive, scruffy and dirty from wintering outside in a part of the world where it rained more days than it didn't, some with horns, some hanging with clarts, most of them showing a ribcage beneath their shaggy coats. It is as much as he can do to walk through the sodden gateway, two or three times the mud closing around his wellington and near sucking it from his foot.

'Away.' With a stick in one hand, he shoos the cows from his path until he reaches a couple of battered troughs, with holes in the end to let the water out. 'Come out the way, ya buggers.'

Once he has sprinkled the food into the troughs he retreats to the gate for a minute or so to let them feed. It would take a lot more than the meal he had offered them to see meat back on their skinny bones. Henry reaches into the back of the Land-rover and lifts out a second sack, fawn brown and unlabelled. Opening it up, he pulls out a severed cow's ear, partly congealed in blood.

'Go on, ma beauties.' He makes his way back into the field and chucks the ear into the feed trough. 'Go on, make the most of it. Summer will soon be here.' He reaches back into the sack again, this time pulling out a cow's hoof. 'Aye, won't be long now!'

4th March 2001

The cattle mart at Carlisle had been around a long time, since it roots began in another century in an old building near the railway station. Replaced in the seventies with a modern structure, the now familiar spot is ideally located near the M6 motorway, and one of, if not the, busiest livestock market in the UK. Two or three days every week of the year, the car and lorry-parks would swell with farmers, breeders, buyers and butchers all of whom used it for regular business. Cleverly designed with its four sale-rings all leading off one central concourse it was also attached to a conference room which in turn housed a pub and restaurant, the latter of which opened into the evenings to serve the local community.

And it was the local community that it was serving this night, not with food but hopefully with information. Situated in the main gateway between England and Scotland, farmers from a radius of 50 miles and more had convened here at the invitation of the government, to be briefed on the latest situation with the foot and mouth crisis, first-hand. Its carpark was now full of Land-rovers and pick-ups, as Nev and Ron arrive, struggling to find a space.

As they enter the conference hall, space was again at premium, as extra seats were brought in to house an audience of well over 200 anxious men and women, with more standing around the walls. At the head of the room a stage had been set up with a long table at which currently sat two men, chief of Agriculture at MAFF, Professor Prince, and a younger man dressed in a tweed sports jacket, who fidgeted with a sheaf of papers and a glass of water while he waited.

At precisely 8 p.m. he taps the microphone, checking it was working before standing to address the crowd. 'Good evening ladies and gentlemen, thank you all for coming this evening. Some of you may know me, my name is Richard Evans and I am chairman of the National Farmers Union. The purpose of this evening's get together is to bring you up to date with the latest on the foot and mouth epidemic, after which we will let you put your questions to the Minister of Agriculture, Ralph Green. As you know, it has been ten days since the first case of the disease was discovered on a pig farm. As of this afternoon, we have since had 142 cases across the country, 72 of which have been in the county of Cumbria. As well as the confirmed cases, a further 222 farms have had their animals culled in an attempt to stop the disease spreading by direct farm contact. I will now hand you over to Professor Prince from MAFF to explain what we are doing to contain the problem. Professor?'

Prince stands to the rostrum, looking nervous. 'Good evening, er, gentlemen. Firstly, the Minister of Agriculture sends his apologies. He has been caught up in traffic so may be a little late.' A few jeers of dissatisfaction ripple through the crowd, halting his words for a couple of seconds. 'As you may be aware, this is a particularly aggressive strain of foot and mouth disease that we are dealing with here and, in some cases, we have seen it mutate. There has been much discussion about using a vaccination to control the disease and I, for one, have been in favour of that route. However, after initial tests of the vaccine being successful in the laboratory, we have found that once the virus has mutated, the same vaccine becomes ineffective in many cases. Hence, we at the Ministry feel that unfortunately vaccine is not the answer....'

Nev's voice rings out from the third row. 'Never mind telling us what you can't do, tell us what you can do!'

The outburst is backed up by a few 'here-here's.

Blatantly ruffled, the professor continues. 'We believe that 90% of the cases we have had have been transferred by contact or by animals in close nasal proximity of each other. Just this morning, the government has approved a new approach to the problem, and that is to extend the radius of the contiguous cull.'

Another voice heckles this time. 'Speak English, man?'

Prince does his best to ignore him. 'That is to say that, as from midnight tonight, we intend to slaughter all animals within the distance of one mile in any direction from a confirmed case of the disease.'

Nev whispers to his pal. 'Bloody hell, Ron. A mile? You're only a mile from me!'

'More personnel are being drafted into the area to help speed up the slaughter process,' Prince continues.

'Aye, more bloody cowboys!' Nev whispers again, before shouting out, 'You need a bloody army, mate!'

'Sir, please don't call out.' Richard Evans stands up, pointing. 'You will have your chance to ask questions shortly.'

Nev sits impatiently while the Professor goes through some more statistics and eventually sits down. Richard stays seated as well, glancing at his watch, then agitatedly speaking from his seat. 'Right, we have time to take a few questions. Unfortunately, the Minister has not managed to make it, but I am sure Professor Prince can quite aptly handle this. Yes, Sir, in the second row.'

One of the farmers stands up and addresses the two men, his face shining under the overhead lights as he speaks. 'Is it true that if we had implemented vaccination immediately, we would have easily contained the spread before the virus got a hold?'

The professor was quick to react to this one, as though he had anticipated the question. 'There may be an element of truth in that and also that it caught us off guard. We certainly didn't have enough vaccine in stock to do the whole country, but we may have had a better chance.'

The questioner wasn't satisfied with this answer. 'Professor, is it also not true that the only reason we didn't use vaccination is that it would have had adverse effects on Britain's export business?'

'No. I don't think our experts ever considered that issue.' Prince is visibly sweating. 'We always had the best interest of the animals in mind.'

Another farmer raises his hand and Richard is pointing at him to allow his question when Nev stands up and butts in. 'Why don't you bring in the army?'

It was a simple question that again Prince was prepared for. 'Our specially trained vets and personnel are handling the situation perfectly well.'

Nev wasn't convinced, raising his voice again. 'Perfectly well? Not from where I am looking. Seems to me they are making a right bollocks-up of it!'

'What makes you suggest that Mr....?'

'Lambert, Nev Lambert. I have worked with your specially trained goons and they are a waste of time. You need some properly trained men!' A mumble of support from the others boosts his confidence. 'And it's not just for the slaughtering. That's the easy bit. What about the carcasses? Isn't it time we put some of them underground?'

'We do have some burial sites in Southern England, and we are considering the possibility of finding a similar site in the North.' Prince was doing his best to plug the gap but even he had no real conviction.

Nev continued, now he had the floor. 'Well, while you are considering it, there are hundreds, maybe thousands of carcasses rotting around the place. That can't be healthy, can it? You need men, proper kit, proper leadership. A military operation. You goons couldn't run a bath, let alone a country.'

'I assure you, Mr. Lambert, we and the government have the situation under control.' Prince is looking around for another person, anyone, who he can converse with to take the spotlight off the embarrassment he is being bombarded with.

Nev takes it as a queue to pipe back down, getting up from his seat and heading outside for a cigarette, still seething. As he leans against the wall in the carpark, his back to the icy wind, a stocky figure in jeans and kagool approaches him. Nev looks him up and down suspiciously so the man feels the need to quickly introduce himself.

'Mr. Lambert. Can I have a word?'

'Sure. What's up?'

The voice is English, Southern, and doesn't quite fit in around this meeting. 'That was a good speech you made in there. My name's Ross Davidson, freelance reporter. I have been putting together a story on the handling of this crisis. Fancy a chat over a pint?'

Nev stubs out his cigarette. 'I guess so.' He follows Ross around the corner and into the Shepherds Inn. The man orders two pints and takes them to an empty table near the back. From his pocket he produces a small tape-recorder and places it on the table next to the beers.

'Don't mind, do you?'

Nev shakes his head. 'Depends what you want to know?'

'You seem to be quite knowledgeable about the slaughter.' Ross asks, matter-of-factly. 'Did you say you had worked for the Ministry?'

'I am not in their regular employ if that's what you mean.' Nev laughs. 'But I have done a few days with them, bunch of clowns that they are. I just thought I had a bit to offer and I need money to feed my family since they laid me off on the trucks.'

'Trucks?'

'I was driving a lorry for Armstrongs....look, what is it you want mate?' Tiredness was arriving now, the stress of it all starting to mount.

'I am just looking for some real people, genuine farmers affected by the disease. So far, I am being stonewalled by the government, but I have it from a good source that there are a few things they aren't admitting.'

Nev scoffs. 'You don't know anything about me.'

'I know you can stand up for yourself. Stand up to the authorities.'

'What makes you so sure? I did that before, didn't get me too far.'

Ross's eyes lit up. 'Care to elaborate?'

Nev glances at the tape recorder on the table. 'Can we turn that off?'

'If you like.' Ross picks it up and flicks a switch.

'Military, wasn't I. I took the King's shilling.'

'How long for?'

'Enough to see some service.' It wasn't a subject Nev wanted to go into. 'Let's just say it didn't work out for me.'

'Go on.'

'Nah. That's it. I did a few terms, saw some action, in the desert. Had a few problems and became a civilian again. Trying to forget it now. So I don't want that splashed all over your paper, OK. It's not common knowledge and I would rather it stayed that way.'

Ross looks him in the eye. 'Sure, if that's how you want it.'

The stare was returned, Nev narrowing his eyes. 'I do.'

Ross takes a pull from the pint. 'That why you are campaigning to get the army involved, so you can re-join?'

'Re-join? Fuck, no!' Nev splutters. 'I just know that the army would be able to sort out this shit. In no time.'

Ross let some silence break the subject, looking around as though checking they weren't being listened to. It was an old journalistic ploy, to make half important news sound more dramatic. He turns back to Nev. 'You know the reason, don't you?'

'Reason?'

'For not bringing in the army?'

Nev considers the question. 'Money, I guess?'

'Not at all. Try again.'

Nev is getting impatient. 'Go on, spill.'

'Blair is running up to an election.'

'So. What's that got to do with it?'

Ross pulls a notebook from his pocket. 'I did some looking into the country's bylaws. If they deploy the armed forces into war, the government isn't allowed to hold an election until it's over.'

'War? Who said anything about a war?'

Ross continues. 'Well, the rules say that if the army is deployed in any military operations, the same applies.'

The penny is starting to drop in Nev's mind. He unravels what he thinks he has just heard. 'So, you are saying that if they send in the army to do this job, the election can't go ahead?'

'Exactly!'

'For fuck's sake.' Nev exclaims, just a bit too loudly. 'That's outrageous!'

'I'm telling you.' Ross pulls a smug grin.

'So basically, the government is hanging us all out to dry while they paddle their own boat?'

The journalist eyeballs him again, confidently. 'Now will you stand up to them?'

'You bet. You got proof?'

'I can get some.'

Nev drains his pint in one go, before nodding his head. 'What do you want me to do?'

A few hours later, Professor Prince sits on a chair in his hotel room, kicking off his shoes and rubbing his tired eyes. He holds a phone to his ear. 'Well, it wasn't an all-round pleasant experience, put it like that, Minister. These farmers up here are pretty passionate about their stock.'

Ralph Green is on the other end, speaking from his home in London. 'They are just locals, Professor. Surely a man of your experience can handle a few uneducated locals?'

'They were asking why you didn't show up, as promised. That's who they all came to see, not me.'

Green's tone is patronising. 'Nonsense, you are the man at the sharp end of this, the one with the answers.'

'The one with his hands tied more like!'

'Now that's enough of that.' The minister snaps. 'We are doing all we can to help. I don't have the time to go running around the land talking to shit-kicking idiots.'

The professor sighs loudly. 'They are still asking about vaccine, but I gave them the line about the virus mutating, as we agreed.'

'Good. And they bought it?'

'I reckon so.' Prince wasn't very convincing. 'But then there were calls for the army to get involved. I said we didn't require that and we were coping but…'

'No 'buts', Prince. No 'buts' and no army. I thought I made that clear. That order comes from the top!'

He hesitates, rubbing his eyes once more. 'Well, I quelled it for now, but demand is growing. We are running out of manpower. Carcasses are mounting up everywhere. And the press are starting to put the pressure on too. There were a few reporters kicking about tonight. I declined to comment to them, said all comms go through your office.'

Green sounds a little more pleased. 'Exactly. My PR people will deal with that side of it. Anything else?'

The vet thinks for a second. 'They didn't react as bad to the extension of the exclusion zones as I thought they would.'

'Good.'

'But then, that brings me on to another problem.'

'Bloody problems.' Green's turn to be impatient. 'I want solutions, not problems, man!

Prince sighs again. 'I think the compensation is getting a little out of hand.'

'What?'

'We appointed a local firm to do the valuations.' Prince checks his notes. 'Hitherman and Hayes in Carlisle.'

'Yes?'

'Well, I think they might be valuing some of the stock too high.'

The minister takes time to answer. 'I suppose that's a good thing. Keeping the farmers on side and all that. Shows we care.'

'The downside to that is that, for some of these farmers, it makes economical sense to get infected.'

'Come again?' Green seeks confirmation. 'Are you saying they want the disease? I thought you said they were passionate about their stock?'

'Oh, most of them are, Sir. But there are a few who would benefit quite nicely from a pay-out, and that's a problem when we are trying to contain the spread.'

'So you are telling me some people are spreading this deliberately?'

Prince back-pedals a little. 'I have no proof. But with all the livestock markets closed, they can't sell their stock. These guys have no other income. We need to look at that.'

The Minister goes back to his bombastic self. 'Don't

talk such bollocks. It's only for a couple of weeks, till we snuff it out. Then everything is back to normal. They get enough subsidy as it is. Are you suggesting we pay them even more to do their job?'

'Is that an option?' asks Prince, hopefully. 'It might help.'

'No, it bloody well isn't. Now, for God's sake, get this thing wrapped up.'

6th March 2001

Not being the most savvy when it comes to computers, it was a friend of Helen's who had set up her laptop with an internet-camera attached. More than a little nervous, Nev is sitting behind it at the kitchen table, wearing a clean shirt. In the corner of the screen he can see a picture of himself which moves jerkily a few seconds after he does.

The TV is on the worktop showing ITV's breakfast television programme, with a glamorous female reporter talking to camera. 'And now to the foot and mouth crisis. Today we have a special link up with a farmer in a highly infected area who has agreed to keep us updated on the situation. Neville Lambert is on a webcam near Dumfries in Scotland. Good morning, Neville - can you hear me?'

Nev takes a deep breath, remembering his manners. 'Good morning, ma'am.' He glances at the TV to see his face appear, the picture much poorer than the one on his laptop. He looks nervous.

'Neville, thank you for joining us. Am I right in thinking you have a flock of pedigree sheep?'

'Yeah.' He clears his throat. 'Yes. That's right, some quite expensive ones. They are due to lamb next week.'

The reporter wears a smile which oozes practiced

concern. 'And how close has the disease been to your farm?'

'Just a few miles away. But it's getting closer.'

Her voice goes into patronising mode, again polished to a shine. 'Oh, my gosh! So you think you might be next?'

Nev stays calm, not rising to the bait, as Ross had pre-warned him. 'I don't see why it should come to us. We have taken all the precautions we can and we are very isolated here.'

The reporter reads from a piece of paper in front of her before looking directly at him again. 'But you are aware that a new law has been passed by the government that says that all animals in a one mile radius of any outbreak have to be destroyed?'

Nev turns his eyes away for a second. 'Yes. I heard that.'

She can't wait to jump at the chance now, although deemed to be impartial, seizing the upper hand. 'Are your stock within this new zone?'

'I'm not sure.'

'If they are, they will all have to be killed, right?'

Nev stays silent until the presenter pushes the point. 'Mr. Lambert? Is that the case? If so, how do you feel about that?'

Despite expecting this question, the reality of it hits home and he tries to hold back his emotions. 'I don't know. OK?' The nerves start to kick in, but he holds his control, knowing it is his turn to fire back a question and turn the conversation. His voice rises. 'What I do know is that the government can sit in London making as many rules as they like, but it will make no difference. It's people we need to sort this out. Lots of them. Trained people.'

The reporter looks surprised but contains herself professionally. 'People? I thought there were lots of people working to stop this disease?'

He's on a mission now, a speech he has rolled out a few times already. 'Not bloody politicians and pen-pushers. Real people. Folks that can do practical things. The countryside is littered with rotting carcasses. Piles of them everywhere.'

'You're referring to the pyres?'

Nev's not missing a beat now. 'Pyres, fires, call em what you will. It isn't you that has to smell the stench, is it? It doesn't reach you townies in bloody London.'

The reporter is visibly rattled and it shows in her voice. 'I assure you, we 'townies', as you refer to us, are equally concerned about animal welfare.'

He senses the insincerity in her and it annoys him. 'Welfare? Animal bloody welfare. Since when has shooting innocent creatures been classed as welfare?'

'Mr. Lambert, I must ask you to tone down your language.' It's obvious she is getting orders in her ear-piece. 'This is live TV, I am sure I don't have to remind you. We have 14 million viewers.'

Nev softens, still with a lot to say and not wanting to be seen as just another angry farmer. 'All I am saying is that, despite what you are being told by the government, the situation is a complete shambles. Every day we get more cases, disease being spread by all sorts of ways, some of it on purpose. Mr. Blair, if you are watching this, I beg you, please. Bring in some decent folks to sort this out now. Send in the army.' He stares unblinkingly at the camera. 'Before it's too late.'

Half-way through his last sentence the words, 'cut, and get him off air' have already been shouted in the presenter's ear, as she closes with: 'Thank you, Neville. And good luck.'

Immediately the screen cuts to a conservative MP, walking through a street full of flag waving crowds. Nev doesn't realise he has been cut off, and continues, his voice rising again. 'And another thing. Why didn't they vaccinate, eh? Tell me that wasn't another of Blair's tactics to hold hands with bloody Europe?'

Helen is standing in the doorway, watching her husband. 'She gone, Nev. They can't hear you now.'

He glances up at her and then the TV screen. 'Can't, or won't?'

10th March 2001

By early March the nights in West Scotland are starting to draw out but somehow the light is sucked out of this one much earlier than it should have been, as a dark cloud of smoke lingers at the base of the hills. It is an eerie sight that Nev is trying to adjust his eyesight to as he heads his old pick-up towards home, down a lane and away from the main road from Carlisle. Rounding a sweeping bend, the cause of the smoke looms from a distance, a yellow glow at the base of a pyre billowing out the rancid smoke. As he nears, the sight of carcasses piled high is enough to turn anyone's stomach, despite him having witnessed it a few times before. He slows as he passes the field gates, seeing two men in white overalls standing watching the flames, one leaning on a fork and the other smoking a cigarette.

He mutters to himself, 'That's it, lads. Earning your wages, I see. Hope you're keeping warm?'

Turning his eyes back to the road just in time, he swerves to avoid a red Land-rover coming in the opposite direction, pushing his own wheels on to the grass. 'Steady on, Tam,' he mutters, seeing his father-in-law at the wheel putting his hand up in acknowledgement.

After another mile he pulls the truck up to his farm gate, eyeing the sign that reads FOOT AND MOUTH

WARNING, KEEP OUT. Glancing around into the dusk, Nev steps down from the pick-up and removes all his clothes, his bare tattooed arms screwing the garments up and putting them into a black bin-liner which he then stuffs behind the gate post. Next, he washes his boots in the bucket of disinfectant using a wooden handled brush and then removes his socks, scrubbing his bare feet and hands. After opening the gate, he jumps back into the vehicle in just his y-fronts, driving it over a large mat which also squelches with disinfectant. Eventually he pulls into his yard, parking the truck away from the house and sheep building.

Helen is waiting for him and starts to laugh.

'What?' he says, innocently.

'Get in here quick, before someone sees you, ya daft brute!' Inside the kitchen she gives him a big hug, and a kiss.

'What's that for?'

Helen can't contain herself. 'We have some good news.'

'We? What? Come on, spill the beans?'

She grins at him. 'Not till you get some clothes on, you look ridiculous!'

'What the bloody hell are you talking about?'

She hugs him again, and then squeezes his bum. 'Get dressed and come see.'

A few minutes later the two of them head outside to the barn, Nev nearly at a run. He counts the seven ewes in the main pen before he sees the eighth one, standing licking a new-born lamb. Nev grabs his wife's hand as the two of them watch mother nature at its finest.

'I can hardly believe it,' he says, finally. 'My first pedigree lambs. This is it, love. This is the beginning of it. This is the future. This is the bloody future, I'm telling you.'

11th March 2001

'We should be there by lunchtime at this rate.' Brian focusses on the motorway ahead, both hands on the wheel. The journey up from Bristol hadn't been the easiest, with roadworks on the M5 which seemed to take up most of the way. Now they were near Worcester it would at least be a clearer run up to Birmingham, especially if they missed the rush hour. He slows a little, pulling the car in behind a short high sided lorry and rubs his eyes. Beside him his wife sits quietly, deep in her own thoughts and looking forward to their few days break in the Peak District. In the back, their son is excited, looking out of the window, taking everything in. It is him who notices it first, a trickle of liquid dripping from beneath the tailboard of the lorry in front. A splash hits the car windscreen.

'Arrghhh! Daddy, what's that?'

His father turns on the windscreen wipers which spread a red smear across the glass.

'Oh, my god. Looks like...' He brakes instinctively.

'Is that blood? It is!' shouts his wife. 'It's coming from that lorry, look!'

As he slows down, another lorry behind him peeps its horn before swinging out and overtaking him. It is a similar one to the one in front, a high sided container painted green. As it passes, the boy can see hooves poking up in the air from above the sides, as a rancid smell comes in through the air ducts into the car.

In another few miles the convoy of three lorries leave the motorway at exit six, taking a main road and then a smaller one deep into the Worcestershire countryside.

12th March 2001

Professor Prince is not happy about being summoned to Whitehall. Over the last few weeks he had been far too busy trying to contain a bushfire that is out of control, and it has left him short of sleep and patience. Now he suspects he is about to get more of the same run-around, as his superiors call the shots from a higher source.

'Happier now, Professor? Everything almost there, eh?' Ralph Green sits opposite, comfortable and confident.

'Almost there, Minister? I am not sure I follow.' The professor follows alright, but not in the direction he needs to go.

Green is actually smiling. 'The site, man. The burial site. It's what you wanted, isn't it?'

'It was one suggestion, Sir, yes.' The chief vet sighs inwardly.

'Suggestion?' The smile is still there, false as it maybe. 'Don't be so modest, man. It was your suggestion, your advice. And we took it. PM was very pleased that you had come up with a solution to the problem. Now we can ship all the carcasses into a big pit, just like you said.'

'But. I only mentioned that in passing. It was just one of the options.'

'Nonsense, man. You asked. We listened.' Green claps his hands. 'Voila!'

Prince chooses his words wisely, 'But, from what I recall I said...'

The Minister doesn't let him finish. 'I recall what you said, and you now have it. Surely, you're not going to start complaining, Professor? '

'Sir, if I may speak. I suggested we dug a pit, Sir, in Devon, to bury the infected animals.'

'Exactly.' Green smiles again.

'But, Sir, what you have provided is an airfield. In Worcester!'

'Devon, Worcester. Same difference. Out there, Professor, to the West. Out in the countryside.'

The Professor fires his first barrel. 'But we have had no cases of foot and mouth in Worcestershire, Sir.' His eyes turn towards his shoes. 'Until now, that is.'

'It's an ideal spot, Professor.' It was quite evident the minister isn't even listening. 'PM decided on the very location himself. Ideal for the motorway. Lots of disused space. Already owned by the government so no need to spend any money. Perfect. No need even to dig a hole. Just tip them all on the tarmac, sheet them over and fence it off for a year or so. Soon everything will be forgotten.'

'Are you saying we take all the carcasses from all over the country to one site in middle England, then pile them up and let them rot?' Prince tries hard not to roll his eyes at the mere suggestion.

Stopping to give it some thought, Green replies.

'Yep. That's pretty much it.'

'But what about the locals. The neighbourhood?'

'Why is it you are so hung up about local people, Professor. It's an RAF base. There are always a few disruptions around a military base. Shouldn't have moved near to it if they didn't like disruptions.'

'But it has been closed for nearly 20 years! And the government....'

Green got more animated. 'Now let's get one thing clear here. I **am** the government. And you are not. You asked, we listened. And we provided. Just make sure you tell everyone, alright? Now go and use what we have just given you and end this thing right now!'

13th March 2001

With nearly two weeks since Nev last went out to work he is getting increasingly agitated sitting at the kitchen table each day, helplessly watching the TV and reading the paper. When the phone rings, the distraction is welcomed.

'Hi Ross, what's the latest?' Nev listens while turning down the TV. 'You are joking, right? You have to be pulling my pisser?'

Ross is doing nothing of the sort. 'No joke, mate. Just had a call from my source. Says they have already started shipping the wagons down there from a farm in Merseyside. It's over 100 miles!'

Nev is shocked but then slightly relieved. 'So, the military are involved then?'

'No, that's just it. Blair is so damned clever he has managed to wangle it. Just some TA and part-timers in uniform on an old military base making it look like he is deploying the services, but he isn't. So, he can still get his election through. You have to admire the guy, even if you don't like him.'

'Admire him?' Nev's distain for the Prime Minister had never been hidden. 'He's a lying shite, and no mistake. Wouldn't want to buy a second-hand car off the bloke, for sure!'

Helen arrives through the kitchen door and raises an

eyebrow.

'You willing to stand up to him in public again?' Ross asks.

'What, back on the telly, you mean?' He glances at his wife, with a half-grin. 'Doubtful they would have me back on there again, I think I upset a few people.'

'No, just in print this time. I think I got a buyer for my story, the Daily Mail want a piece of it.'

'And you want to use my name, right?' Nev picks up a cup of tea Helen has just set down in front of him. 'Ta!'

'Can I?' Ross is asking, expectantly.

'What's in it for me?

'You want money? Or you want to make a difference? Don't think you can have both.'

'Well some cash would come in handy right enough. Things are a bit tight round here just now. What do you mean - 'make a difference?'

Ross sighs at the other end of the phone. 'This story, it's all about exposing the government, bringing them down, even.'

'Now wait a minute.' Nev's reaction lifts his voice a notch. 'I am not going to get involved in your political wrangles, I got enough on my plate without upsetting the cart...but…'

The journalist buts in. 'Don't worry, I've got plenty of back-up on that score. No, I would just like you to verify what we have talked about. You know, about this disease still spreading because it's not been handled properly.'

Again, Nev looks at his wife, raising a quizzical eye. 'Well, I suppose...'

'It will just take five minutes of me asking you a few questions.'

Nev sits down. 'Aye, go on then.'

15th March 2001

The ewe with the two lambs is now grazing in the field. Nev stands at the gate and gazes at them, surprised how fast they have grown in just a few days. He catches sight of his pal, Ron, opening the farm gate and washing his boots in the bucket, before entering. Ron makes his way to the field gate and shakes Nev's hand. Nev smiles at him. 'How you doing, mate?'

'Aw, you know. Mustn't grumble.' Something in Ron's eye suggests he could grumble plenty.

Above them, the sky greys over and Nev glances up. 'I see you didn't take my advice and get away from this bloody weather?'

'Nah. It's not me, Nev, that sunshine lark. Not happy unless I got my oilskins on!' Ron looks at the ewe and lambs. 'Bloody hell, mate, that's a bonny pair. Some arse on that tup lamb!'

'You reckon they're OK then?"

'More than OK.' Ron nods 'And she seems to be feeding them alright?'

'Oh aye. Got bags of milk.'

'They pair will need it too. Couple of strong lambs like that'll soon have her dry. You've done the right thing getting her out into the paddock for the day though.'

Nev acknowledges the compliment from the more experienced farmer. 'I'll give her another 10 minutes then she can go back inside out the rain. He turns towards the house. 'Come on in, Helen's got the kettle on, if you've got time.'

Ron replies, 'I've plenty of that just now. But I came here to bring you this. Have you seen it?' He hands Nev a rolled-up newspaper from inside his jacket.

'Made the paper then, did I?' Nev smiles.

'Aye, page three. You might not like it though.'

Opening the roll, Nev looks at the page to see himself standing there, a grainy photograph of him in army uniform. 'Bloody hell. How did they find all that out? I never told him this stuff. Bastard says I was kicked out the forces. I was never kicked out.' He continues looking at the piece as they headed to the house.

Half an hour later, he is pacing the kitchen, mobile phone in his hand. His wife sits and watches him. She knows there is little she can say when he is in a mood like this, but she tries. 'It's just a newspaper scandal. Don't let it get to you, Nev.'

Nev shakes his head, ignoring her. 'Bloody answerphone again.' He listened to the end of Ross's voice saying leave a message, and then raises his own. 'At least have the decency to return my calls, you cowardly bastard!' He ends the call, red faced.

'Calm down Nev, please.' She tries again.

Instead of calming down, Nev picks up a can of

strong lager and takes a long swig. 'I thought I was helping. Making things right. And all he has done is chucked me under the bus, just to sensationalise his story. It just isn't fair, Helen. I'm telling you.'

Helen quietly finishes reading through the article again before replying

'It's not all bad, Nev. He makes some pretty good accusations in here about the government. And you are only a small part of it.'

'Disgraced soldier, lorry driver and small-time farmer stands up to Prime Minister! Only part of it, yeah? Only the bloody scapegoat part of it, you mean.'

She stands up, still trying to comfort him. 'It's just an angle, Nev. Newspapers do it all the time. Little guy takes on big guy, that's what sells papers.' The phone rings, which makes her jump. She answers it sternly. 'No, he's not here at the moment. And no, I won't bloody comment.' Her face is flushing now. 'Vultures, the lot of them.'

Nev can see she is annoyed too and sits down, reading the article again himself. 'Well, if he is right about Blair not bringing in the army because of the election, he certainly has stirred up a shit storm.' He takes another swig of beer. 'I certainly have stirred up a shit storm. Even if they have all my military background mixed up. I'll be branded as a troublemaker for ever after this. I bet even Armstrongs will fire me now. If I have a job to go back to. That bastard sure has stuffed the knife into me good and proper.'

The sound of the kitchen clocks ticks away the silence for over a minute. Helen eventually breaks it. 'Well, Nev. It's up to you now. You have been put in the firing line. You can either run or stand and fight. I know you, darling, and I love you. And I know which one you will choose.'

He nods slowly, without looking at her. 'Aye, you do. And I thought my fighting days were over. Well, seeing as I am in the shit already, I might as well stand up and say my piece.'

Nev spends much of the afternoon out with the sheep, bringing the ewe and her lambs into the barn and then sitting watching them, urging one of the others to lamb to take his mind off things. By the time it gets dark his mind is made up and he makes his way back to the house, announcing his is off to the pub.

Within a couple of hours, he is standing on the doorstep, fuelled by at least three pints of beer. In front of him are an assembled throng of reporters as a spotlight shines in his face. He looks through the night at them and clears his throat.

'Uh, thanks for coming. Or for tracking me down at least. You may have read some shit - I mean - dirt - about me in the national paper so I want to put the record straight. Firstly, yes, I was in the army for three years, but I left of my own accord, OK. Sure, we had a few disagreements, but it was my choice to go - I was NOT thrown out!'

A brash reporter fires a question. 'So why did you leave, Neville?'

'That information is not relevant, and it is personal, so I am not here to talk about it. I just want to set the record straight on this,' he holds up the newspaper article, 'and then move on to that mess.' He indicates to smoke billowing from a pyre in the distance. More questions are asked which he ignores, and some reporters are writing things down, as he continues. 'I was approached by one of you to give my opinion on the foot and mouth crisis.' He scans the crowd of a dozen or so, looking for Ross, who unsurprisingly isn't there. 'Me, just an ordinary hard-working bastard, trying to have a go at making a life! He made quite a meal of it so now I am in the papers.' He pauses to light a cigarette, blowing the smoke out into the night so it causes a haze in the spotlight. 'My opinion may not be worth much but, being as I am in the news, you might as well hear it in full. I can't say I speak for everyone in the farming community, but I have a few chaps behind me who share my beliefs.' Behind him a few men shuffle into view, including Ron. 'As farmers in the North of the country, we believe the government doesn't care a hoot about our wellbeing and livelihood. As far as they see, the country stops at Watford!' This creates a few sniggers behind him, and a cough from the crowd out front. He continues, getting back into his stride. 'As mentioned in the story by this reporter,' he holds up the Daily Mail, 'we have suggested that the only way to handle this crisis, which is now completely out of control, is to bring in the army. I have said it two or three times and at last a few people are listening. It needs to be done and to be done NOW! Mr. Blair, if you are listening, please act now and delay your general election!'

A reporter shouts out. 'I thought they had already deployed the military?'

'No, they haven't.' Nev snaps back at him. 'That site down in England is just a smoke screen. Smoke and mirrors, that is a trait of this government, and especially of this Prime Minister. The men working on that site and driving these lorries full of infected carcasses are just volunteers. These men need back-up, direction, leadership and power to act for the good of the country as a whole, not just for the good of London.'

The reporter is glad of the attention and probes again. 'Are you volunteering to lead them, Neville?'

Nev laughs out loud which extends into a coughing fit. 'Me? Christ, no. It needs a fully qualified and experienced officer. Someone with a high rank to control the whole shebang.'

'What would you do, if you were that person?' comes a shout from the night.

He considers his answer while others fire even more questions, overlapping each other. 'What would I do? Well for a start, I would base operations up here in the North, where the real problems are. I would need machines, lots of them. Great big ones like we used in ... like they use in war zones. Then we need some land to work on, somewhere accessible, near a main road network. And then, in my opinions, we need to dig a bloody great big hole!'

17th March 2001

Gerald Priestly had trained to be an accountant at college for a couple of years before he changed tack and took a job with the Merchant Navy. For a good few years he toured the world and had firsthand experience with the shipping trade, including import and export. Having been born in rural middle England, on his return to UK, he opted for further North and an office job with a small building firm. It was there he met his wife, Alison, who ran the sales desk. After just three years they decided to make a go of business for themselves and put all their savings into a farmyard which they subsequently developed into a garden centre, complete with cafe and farm shop. Jardleys, as it was called, was ideally placed near the A7 exit for Gretna Green and traded as much with tourists as it did with locals. For over ten years it had grown and prospered - until now that is. What would normally be a full carpark, even in springtime, contained just two cars, his and his wife's.

Gerald is on the phone while his wife sits opposite him typing on a PC keyboard. Behind her some plants sit in large pots, as though watching their own fate. 'I know I said Friday, Richard, but I need more time to raise the capital. This damn disease has pretty much dried us up. I have thrown all my own cash at it already, but I am hoping we can canvass some family money. Can you give me another two weeks?' The caller isn't buying it, so he starts to plead. 'No? Well, how long then?'

Alison looks sadly at him, fearing the answer.

'Two days?' he says, quietly. 'OK, I'll do my best.' He ends the call and looks across at his wife who has stopped typing. 'Bank needs thirty grand in two days, or we are done.'

He stands now, his brow sweating, and looks out of the window at the empty carpark, a tear welling in his eye.

'I am so sorry, love.' His wife concedes. 'You did all you could.'

He looks her in the eye. 'I guess it's time to send out that email, eh?'

Priestly walks through the door and down amongst the plants, his portly frame stopping to touch one. At the main door, he pulls a CLOSED sign across and sits on a flower pot, head in hands.

At the other end of the country, in central London, the man responsible for all facets of agriculture for the whole of Great Britain is having a conversation with his boss, the man in charge of the nation.

'Yes, Tony. I know that is what you said but this thing just won't go away.'

Tony Blair is not happy. 'What about this bloody irritating pipsqueak, shouting his mouth off to the press. I thought I told you to bury that?'

'I put Murdoch on to it, Sir. He dug up some dirt to discredit the lad, something to do with going AWOL from the forces. I thought that would do the trick, but he seems to have the backing of several farmers from the North West, as well as a few local businesses. They are all pointing to the same solution.'

'*They* are pointing?' Blair raises his voice uncharacteristically, 'It's not up to them to point, Nicholas. We do the pointing and they look where we tell them, that's how it works. And right now, we are looking at a 52% majority in five week's time. That means, Nicholas, we all keep our jobs for another four years. So whatever propaganda your soldier man is spouting about, put an end to it. We have thrown in a few extra mill, and you have your burial site and your team of lackies.'

Green backs down, spluttering, 'Yes, Sir. But the stats are going against us. 450 cases and rising 20% per day. Three-to-four-day backlog on shifting the dead animals. Two-to-three weeks cleaning up the farms after they have gone. New cases popping up in previously non-affected areas. I emailed the report to your office this morning.'

But the Prime Minister is no longer listening to reason. 'Do you really think I have time to read every bloody report that comes in? Especially now? We are fighting a fight here. And we are going to win. So don't you dare let your statistics screw up our chances. Fix the damn things. Spin it, man. Make them say what we want them to hear. Good god, man, we don't keep Murdoch in sweets for nothing! Put him to work!'

That same evening, the subject of work was also on the minds of a small farmer and his wife, as the money situation started to pile up along with the bills. Nev lies on his back in bed, looking at the ceiling as the radio plays in the background.

'It won't be for long, pet. You can cope. Just a few days away and a chance to earn some decent money. We need money, Helen. And at least this way I don't have to shoot anything. Just a few days work down south.'

Helen is propped up on one elbow. 'I am heavily pregnant, Nev, in case you hadn't noticed? I can't manage the kids, and a job, and your sheep on my own.'

He is expecting this reaction and stays cool. 'I have thought about that, and that's why I have asked me Mam to come and stay.'

Expectedly that changes the mood. 'Your Mum? Nev, your Mum has never been on a farm in her life!'

He still focuses on the ceiling. 'Maybe. But she can look after you. Great cook, our Mam. And she can look after the children. Great with children.'

Helen laughs. 'Yes and look how you turned out!'

'What do you mean, like?' He grins now, knowing the worst is over, for now, anyway. 'I am a fine upstanding member of the community. Never upset no one!'

Right on cue, Blair's voice can be heard on the radio.

'Aye.' She replies. 'Except him, maybe?'

Nev turns up the radio to listen to the PM who is giving a news conference.

'...everything is under control. Number of cases is decreasing every day and we are catching up with clearing the backlog since we put more resources on.'

A reporter shouts out in the background, a voice Nev thinks he recognises. 'Are you going to postpone the election Mr. Blair?'

The PM stays calm, polished as always. 'And why would we do a thing like that?'

Nev can't contain himself as the radio goes back to the newsreader. 'Number of cases slowing down? Not round here, mate. And as for the backlog, you want to drive down the Gretna road and smell it.' He fumbles with the knob to turn the sound down and then turns to Helen, giving her a kiss. 'I'll be away at first light, pet. Mam will be at Dumfries station at 11.30. I'll check the yows before I go and call you later.'

18th March 2001

'People come in all shapes and sizes,' thought Helen, as she watches the train begin to unload its cargo of passengers. There are men in grey and tweed, kids in bright colours, women looking tired. Through the crowd one woman stands out, if only for her smile, peroxide and girth. She is carrying two large bags, quite well balanced for a woman in her fifties in heels that height.

Helen greets her with a hug, attempting to take the bags from her. 'Hello Pam, let me help you with that?'

'What in your condition?' Her voice is as coarse as rolled oats. 'Don't be so daft, girl.' She indicates to Helen's midriff. 'That's my grandchild you got in there, and it best stay in there. For now, any roads.'

A little taken aback, Helen tries not to let it show as she engages in conversation whist walking towards the exit. 'How was your trip, Pam?'

Quick to take the stage, Pam recounted her journey. 'Too hot! Why do they always make those carriages so hot? Like a bloody furnace in there. Nearly had to strip off naked!' The grin is as natural to her as rain to the hills. 'Wouldn't be the first time, eh?'

Helen blushes slightly, smiling politely at the joke and wondering about the days to come. 'Car's this way.

Only a few yards. You sure you can manage both bags?'

'Don't you worry about me, lass.' The older woman replies sternly. 'Been managing on my own for 20 years! Bags, boxes, brooms, kids, everything. Just about everything.' She pauses, producing that grin again. 'Except men!'

Her breathing is quite heavy as they reach the car, lifting her bags into the boot and taking the passenger seat. She turns to Helen, looking her in the eye. 'Anyway, enough about me.' Her tone softens. 'How are you, chick? You bearing up OK? My Nev keeping you right, is he?'

'He does OK but he is a bit stressed at the moment.' Helen starts the engine. 'This disease thing is starting to wear him down. Wear us all down.'

'You can say that again. I saw him, on the telly. Our Nev, standing right there, proud as punch. Reminded me of his father, till he buggered off to London. Bastard!'

Helen looks straight ahead, chewing at her lip. She decides it is best not to answer the woman. Let her get it said, so they can move on.

Not that Pam would let her get a word in anyway. 'Looked as thin as a pin, did Nev. Don't you feed the lad? Not hard to feed, our Nev. Used to eat everything I put in front of him. Doesn't he like your cooking? Chips. He likes chips. Loves em.'

Holding her breath for a few seconds, she stares out at a red traffic light, momentarily screwing up her eyes shut before speaking. 'It's just stress, Pam. We all get it, but he is under a lot of pressure just now, what with the sheep, the kids, no job, this problem.'

Pam isn't buying that. 'Stress, my arse! I brought up four kids on my own, with one hand tied behind my back. You only got a couple, and a husband to help. A few sheep can't take much looking at.'

This went unanswered, for the remainder of the journey.

By early evening, the air has cleared a bit, as well as the furniture which has been re-arranged to accommodate a mother-in-law's temporary requirements. Lunch had been and gone, when Pam had almost force fed her some tinned soup. Now she enters the kitchen carrying Sophie and looking a bit more relaxed. George follows behind her.

'Did you bring me a present, Granny Pammy?'

Helen stops him. 'George, don't be so rude!'

But Pam just smiles. 'Well, I might just have something for you, young man.' She pulls out a chocolate bar from her bag and hands it to him.

'Er.' Helen goes to intercept it. 'We don't normally give him chocolate, Pam. Makes him hyper.'

'Rubbish. All kids love chocolate. It's their favourite.'

'I didn't say he doesn't like it, it's just that we don't give it to him.'

Ten minutes later the phone rings, by which time George is charging around the room making sheep noises as loud as he can. Pam has settled down to watch Coronation Street on TV, the volume turned up high.

Helen picks up the phone. 'Oh, hi love. Thought it might be you.' She listens for a second before replying. 'Yes, she arrived a few hours ago. With chocolate and enough luggage to stay a month!' She covers the receiver with her hand. 'George, be a bit quieter darling, please. Daddy's on the phone.'

George ignores her, making more sheep noises and charges out into the kitchen.

Nev is amused. 'Sounds like you brought the flock indoors, luv? How they doing?'

Helen moves out into the hallway so she can keep an eye on the boy and out of earshot of Pam. 'They are doing fine, Nev. Nothing to report, really. Lambs sucking OK, and I am sure they have grown since this morning. No sign of the others lambing yet. So all fine, really. My Dad said he might drop in tomorrow. Just for a look. You don't mind, do you?'

Nev sighs. 'I suppose not.'

'Anyway, how's your day?'

'Not much happening today,' he replies, sounding bored already. 'Managed to get booked into a small pub called The Red Lion with the other lads. Will get a couple of pints tonight, and then away early. Got a sharp start in the morning. Speak tomorrow, eh?'

Once they have said their goodbyes, Nev steps back inside, stubbing out a cigarette on the step and goes through a door to a crowded bar. He makes his way to the bar and takes a high stool. Behind it a tall attractive brunette makes the usual bar-maid conversation. 'Chilly out there, eh? Another pint?' Her brogue is Irish, soft and sexy.

Nev nods a cheeky smile. 'Got any other suggestions to warm me up?'

She has his measure already. 'You can try the local brew if you want. Served warm and you'll run to the toilet that many times it'll soon get the blood flowing again.'

Nev laughs out loud. 'You're not exactly selling it to me. I was more thinking of a dram of something peaty.'

The laugh is a bit too flirtatious. 'Ah, that old trick. Get the bar maid to reach up to the top shelf so you can see her knickers, eh?'

'Uh. I was…'

She laughs even louder. 'I was just kidding. Which one you want?'

He blushes slightly. 'The cheapest will be fine.'

The barmaid opens a bottle of Grouse and pours a measure. As she does so he is studying her while her back is turned and she catches him in the mirror but says nothing. When she puts it in front of him and starts pouring a lager as well, he starts the chat. 'Not from around here, are you?'

'Me? That's rich coming from you.' Her Irish accent toned down a notch. 'Reckon I am more local than...let me think. North. Cumbria somewhere?'

'Aye. Carlisle.' He nods, 'You?'

'Dublin.' She says walking away down the bar. Her eyes glow with beauty as she teases him again, vaguely waving towards the window and grinning. 'It's over there, somewhere.'

Nearly four hours later, during which Nev has read the national paper, the local paper and most of the beer mats on the bar, he studies his pint, and glances at the only other customer left in the cosy bar, an old man sitting by the fire, half asleep.

The girl finishes clearing a table and approaches him, 'It's Siobhan, by the way.' She takes the next stool and crosses her legs. Nev watches them, his mind starting to whirr with drink. Her tone is friendly as she nudges his ribs. 'Wanna tell me about it?

Nev looks up. 'How long you got?'

'About a minute and a half till I chuck you outside.'

'Outside? But I'm staying here,' his protests waking the old man by the fire.

'That's 30 seconds,' muses Siobhan, 'clock's ticking!'

'Which bit you want to hear?'

The girl sighs. She's been here many times before. 'Aw, I dunno. The wife at home, troubles at work, sexual frustration. You chose.'

'What's this. Kiss and tell?'

'Nice try, buster. You got about 40 seconds left!'

'Okay, okay.' Nev nods. 'Yes. Troubles at work. You don't want to hear it.'

'I'm asking, ain't I?' Her tone is genuine but he decides to remain silent, so she continues, stating what she knows already. 'You're with the other guys, aren't you? The slaughter troopers. But you don't fit in with em do you? You're too good for that job? How am I doing?'

Nev lights a cigarette, offering her one.

'Nah, I quit.'

'When?'

She grins. 'Just about every week?'

They both laugh which seems to break the deadlock. Nev feels himself relaxing in this company, his guard dropping. 'Yeah, guess you got me sussed. Fish outta water here. Not my kinda bag, cleaning up a shitty mess. Don't get me wrong, I don't mind getting my hands dirty. It's just I don't like cleaning up other folk's stuff, that's all. Wasn't brought up that way. Don't mind clearing up after myself. Even make my own bed, you na.' He lets out another laugh. 'Even make the wife's bed, sometimes.'

'Ex-military, right?'

He nods again. 'Shows, does it?'

'Let me think.' She's teasing again, but dangerously close to the mark. 'Loner. Doesn't fit in easily. Troubled mind. Can make a bed. Yep, forces, fer sure. Seen action, probably?

'Don't want to talk about it.'

'You sure?'

He looks into her eyes, irresistibility taking control. 'Thought you were kicking me out in the snow?'

She breaks his gaze. 'One, it's not snowing. Two, you live upstairs anyway. And three. Well, I haven't worked bars for ten years not to know the difference between a guy who wants to get something off his chest and a guy who wants to get on to mine. And you're the former, buddy. So out with it.'

His attempt is just a bit too half-hearted. 'Shouldn't we just go to bed instead? Much less boring.'

'What? Together? No, sir.' She sighs loudly for effect. 'Married! Look?' before pointing to his left hand. 'Wedding ring. See?'

'Aw, damn, I near forgot.'

Instead of throwing him out, Siobhan stands up and goes behind the bar, pours two whiskies, and sets one down in front of each of them, before sitting back down.

'Right Neville, start talking. I'm all ears.'

'You know my name?'

'It's tattooed, right there on your forearm,' the smile is back, 'dumb ass!'

From there, Nev's world turned itself inside out as he closed his eyes. He could hear himself speaking but the view was a cinema reel of history, a place he knew so well, but somewhere he very rarely went.

A young Nev is catching a Stagecoach bus in a quiet bus station, chucking in his bag and taking a seat. Shortly he is signing a form and then getting a haircut.

'Left school at 16. Got in a spot of bother with a few local bobbies. Probation. Usual stuff. No excuses.'

Next a bunch of army lads are running along an assault course, an officer yelling at them.

'It was the probation officer's idea that I join up, see the world. Get away for a while until I grew up a bit. Me Mam wasn't so keen. Think she expected me to stay home and pay her bills. But I never really questioned it, just headed off one Saturday. They say the training is tough, but it never bothered me too much. Just a quick way of getting fit. Soon settled in to a daily routine and they don't shout at you too much if you do things the right way. To some of the lads nine years seemed like a life sentence but I never saw it that way. Just something to do, keep me occupied like. First six months soon went by.'

Now he is now in the forest in camouflage kit, rifle in hand, wide eyed and looking for something to shoot at.

'I'd never fired a rifle before but somehow it felt easy. Just a quick aim and I hit the target pretty much every time. They said I was a natural.'

The vision changes, now he is bailing out of a Hercules aircraft, behind a dozen other parachutists.

'Said they needed lads with skills down there in the desert. I'd never been south of Penrith before, so a stint in the sun seemed quite inviting. Not that I was in a position to argue. A few months sitting around drinking local beer, keeping the peace and keeping my head down, that's what the other lads said.'

He's on his belly, crawling along in sand.

'Next thing I know, a lot of guys in tea-towels are fighting a whole lot of other guys in tea-towels over the price of oil and we are stuck in the middle. As I saw it, the war in the Gulf was pretty straight forward, one country invading another to nick their oilfields. Oil they believed was rightfully theirs due to some historic claims. If they'd been left to get on with it, it would have been over in a year or so and everything back to normal.'

President George Bush Snr is inspecting troops and then appears to be giving a speech to the ranks.

'Except the Yanks had different ideas. George Bush waving his dick around, in the name of humanity issues. War-mongering bastard couldn't wait to get Arab blood on his hands and of course he got all the encouragement he needed from the senate, who had another agenda. It didn't take a mastermind to work out that they just wanted in on the control of world oil supplies. Next thing John Major is wading in, promising back-up support, and my arse goes on the line for him, stirring up a shit-storm that neither he, nor anyone, could ever win. But, back then, I was as brainwashed as the rest of them into believing we were doing the right thing by forming a coalition army.'

Amongst the darker caves on the hillside over a mile away, the crosshairs meet on a man sitting cross-legged with an AK47 rifle in his hand. Beneath the chequered agal around his head, Nev sees the face of a young teenager, possibly no more than 14.

The silence is deafening.

'They gave me a job. A very specific job. Get in close. Then hide and wait. Shoot when they are not expecting it. Pick em off one at a time.'

Nev is hiding out in an old burned out building, Arab soldiers running around in the streets, occasional gunfire.

'So, that's what I did. For a few months. Living on my own, eating stale rations, and whatever else I could find. Hiding from the enemy. And from those fucking Scud missiles that kept raining in overhead. I was hardly going to win a war single handedly, but I felt I was making a difference, For once in my life. So I stuck at it, enjoyed it almost.'

In his mind, Nev watches himself being pulled out of a ditch at gun point by two Iraqi soldiers.

'As a kid, I was pretty good at hide and seek. This was a game I could play, no problem. Began to believe I was invisible. But I got lazy, didn't I? In hindsight it was pretty obvious they would be looking for me, since I had been picking off their people through the dark like a coward. One day I stayed too long in the same place.'

Nev opens his eyes, drains the whisky glass, closes them again and retreats back into his own head, as though hypnotised.

In the back of an army truck, two Iraqi soldiers sit either side of him conversing in Arabic. He is bleeding and beaten up, hardly recognisable. When the vehicle goes over a bump, he groans but they ignore him.

'I never considered myself a lucky person. Just an ordinary guy doing extraordinary stuff, best I could. My own fault I got caught. In fact, I just thought this was the end and that somehow, in a strange way, I deserved to die. To be punished for what I had done. Punished for doing a job for which I was paid the King's shilling. Die for my country, like so many others had before me. The beating that I took that morning was enough to kill most men. I was barely alive. I suppose that's the difference between what I did and what those guys wanted. I killed. One shot, bang, job done. They didn't want that, they wanted revenge and it required suffering. Suffering and pain. No, I never considered myself lucky.'

A Toyota Land-cruiser driving along, suddenly hits a land mine and the front wheel explodes, sending the truck off the track where it turns on its side. The driver is killed, and the two men thrown from the back. Nev is thrown out too, all three lying on the ground.

'No, I never considered myself lucky, until that afternoon. There was no God to help me. No higher being to save me. Just myself, and a slim chance of clutching life from certain death.'

In his frame he sees himself stumble to his feet and grab a rifle near the burning vehicle. He points it to one of the captors and fires a single shot. It hits the man between the eyes. Then he does the same with the other two before toppling over on the ground again, unconscious. The vehicle explodes.

'And one thing you learn from a life like mine.'

A Jeep arrives along the road, flying a US flag. Pan out to see some tanks and armoured vehicles spread out in a line across the desert. The jeep stops and checks the bodies. Nev is still breathing, just.

'You gotta take that chance when it comes. And that, if luck comes your way, one day there might be a price to pay.'

Siobhan speaks for the first time in ten minutes. 'So, you spend the rest of your life looking over your shoulder, that it?'

'Something like that.' Nev stands up, and heads towards the door, stops and turns back.

'Everyone gets it in the end. We all live on a set of scales. No such thing as luck, just good and bad shit in equal measures.' He nods. 'G'night.'

'See ya.' Siobhan gets to her feet and gathers the glasses up. 'Well, aren't you a cheery soul?'

19th March 2001

Ralph Green looks up when he hears a knock on the door of his wooden panelled office. The man who enters has an air of superiority about him that unnerves Green a little. Tall, well groomed and in his fifties, Brigadier Robert Hardcastle had earned the respect of many, but he wasn't a government man.

'Brigadier, please sit down.'

'Minister. How can I be of help?' He brushes an imaginary speck of dust from his khaki trousers.

'That is a question I was rather hoping you could answer for me.' Green says, expectantly.

Hardcastle looks him directly in the eye. 'You sound a little desperate, Minister. If I recall correctly, we spoke seven days ago and you denied requiring help of any kind, except for 'borrowing' some of our military vets and a few trucks.'

'That was then, Brigadier.' Green wipes his brow. 'That was then, and this is ...'

The Brigadier wasn't about to play games. 'This is, if you don't mind me pointing out, an outright shambles. Fifty cases of the disease per day, thing still spreading like wildfire. Nation up in arms. PM in a spin. How am I doing?'

Green is physically rattled. 'I don't need a lecture from you, thank you. I just need a plan, and a budget.'

'You would need to speak to the Minister of Defence about budget.'

'Oh, believe me I have.' Confidence returned to the Minister. 'It's on the verge of being cleared.'

Previously briefed on the situation, Brigadier Hardcastle started to outline a plan he had already formed. 'Firstly logistics. You need a logistics coordinator in place, possibly two.'

'We have all that being run from Page Street in London.'

'With the greatest respect, Minister, I am not sure it is possible to run a rural operation from a city centre HQ. You need a set-up in the affected areas. Men, maps, phones, computers. People with experience in moving things around cleanly and efficiently.'

'Go on.'

Hardcastle is studying a map on the desk. 'Somewhere here. And here.'

Green follows his finger on the map to Dumfries. 'But that's in Scotland. We can't start funding projects north of the border. It will cause all sorts of complications.'

The Brig raises his eyes to the ceiling, then raises his voice. 'Look, it is politics that have gotten you into this mess, Minister. So let's just try and see past the why and focus on the how and where, eh?'

Green stands up. 'Now you look here. You might be used to bossing your troops around, Hardcastle, but I am a Cabinet minister. You cannot talk to me like that.'

The Brigadier is unmoved, speaking slowly, a slight

tone of sarcasm creeping in. 'You wanted my help, and now you have it. So let's not get bogged down with personal issues, shall we.'

An hour later, the same room is now filled with six other men in uniform. A large map is pinned on the wall as the Brig speaks. 'The northern co-ordinator will map out all farms in the area, affected and otherwise. He will be in control of all movements of animals, vehicles and personnel from now on. Nothing north of Liverpool happens without his say so.'

On a central table a to-scale model of the North West of England is spread out, with model trucks and plastic fires. Six army soldiers, men and women, are looking and working on it. A big X is drawn over the town of Wigton.

'Once, and only once, we have assessed the situation, we will make a decision where to bury the dead.'

He looks around at each of the officers in turn, before speaking again. 'Then we will need some recruits, chosen by ourselves. Men with experience, who are ready and willing to stop this thing, rather than just to line their own pockets.'

That same evening, in the area that was being discussed 200 miles away, Pam is feeding the baby at the table while Helen washes dishes. The TV is on, showing 6 o'clock news headlines. She turns it up to hear the presenter. 'The government has today announced that it intends to delay the General Election planned for May 3rd and a new date has been set for June 7th. Reasons given for the postponement are that, with much of the country closed down due to biosecurity measures put in place to help stop the spread of foot and mouth disease, it may not be possible for everyone to get out to the polling stations. Other events, such as April's Cheltenham's Gold Cup Festival have also been postponed or cancelled as the crisis now enters its fourth week and shows no sign of abating. Our reporter in Whitehall has more.'

The footage cuts to a reporter standing in Downing Street with Number 10 in the background. 'An announcement from Number 10 came this morning at 9am, quite out of the blue. It appears that the Prime Minister has done a u-turn on the subject of the election date. However, the reasons that have been put forward suggest that he has been listening to the general public, and particularly the rural sector, in wanting to make sure everyone has an equal opportunity to vote.'

20th March 2001

The North West is not the most densely populated area of Great Britain and parts of it have always suffered from lack of employment. Judging by the queue outside a temporary building set up in the car-park at Carlisle livestock market, a few new jobs around here would be welcome, despite the circumstances. Men are chatting away as though they were waiting for a roller coaster ride rather than a job in the killing fields. Nev has no illusions about what he is expecting, having already witnessed some of it. Although he recognises some of the men, he keeps his thoughts to himself.

As the queue draws nearer, he can see through the window into the makeshift office. Two uniformed army officers are sitting behind a long desk, one male, one female, giving the interviews, one of them leafing through some papers while a man stands agitatedly in front of them.

'I am not sure if you have got the experience we need for this job,' the officer says. 'We are looking for digger and truck drivers, or people with slaughter experience.' He puts the man's paper into a basket on the desk. 'We will keep you on file for now, and if anything else comes along, we have your details. Thank you Mr. Robson.'

The female soldier follows the man to the door, lets him out and nods to Nev. 'Next!'

He steps inside and hands over a sheet of paper containing his resume, before taking a seat and waiting. He's been here before, a long time ago. The officers both look at it for a short while before the male one speaks again. 'A military man, I see. Well ex-military. Looks like they could have done with you on the culling team, Mr. Lambert. We are looking for drivers just now, men with experience. I suppose you would have learnt some of that your army career.'

'I can drive just about anything with wheels. Or tracks, come to that. Did a stint with the tank boys in Iraq. Did all sorts of things, out there.'

The female officer is typing some details into a laptop. Nev sees her eyes change as she stops and shows something to her colleague. He speaks for her, 'Says here you got a commendation, and were offered promotion, Mr. Lambert.'

'Aye, commendable job eh? Shooting folks from a distance.'

The man takes that as an insult. 'It also says you refused the promotion and were quite insolent about it. Is that you, Mr. Lambert? Insolent? A troublemaker perhaps? Haven't I seen you on TV recently?'

Nev sighs. 'Aye, but I wasn't making trouble, just getting you boys a job.'

'And now you want me to give you one. Despite what it says here?'

'I don't know what it says there. I didn't take the promotion because I didn't want to stay, OK?' He is careful not to appear aggressive. He needs this job, they both know that. 'I sustained enough injuries to have the choice of medical discharge. At least two doctors told me that.'

'So I see, but the military doctor said differently?'

Nev declines to reply and the room is silent for a while.

The officer isn't done yet. 'Well, I am not too sure we want trouble in the ranks, Mr. Lambert.'

'Look. I was in the army, and I left, OK? The last thing I want to do is sign back up again. But I do need a job, and I am a good worker, with all the experience you need.' He runs his hands through his hair. Make or break time. 'Christ! It was partly due to me that you guys got in on this. Because I thought you could make a difference and get this thing sorted. All I want to do is bloody help, not be promoted to Colonel! God knows, I am better than most of those goons out there.'

The two officers look at each and then back through the paperwork. Slowly the male officer lifts up a stamp and presses it on to a document. He hands it to Nev. 'OK. Start Monday. We will call you with more details in the next couple of days. In the meantime, I assume you will continue with the job you are currently working on.'

Its early evening before Nev gets back to his digs at the Red Lion Inn. Siobhan sees him come in, and smiles. 'Hey, how'd it go, soldier?'

'Don't ask?

'Not well then.'

'Oh, they gave me a job alright, after the Spanish inquisition.' The two lock eyes for a second too long.

'Start next week.'

'So you'll be leaving us then? Where you headed?'

She puts his pint on the bar, flirting with him.

'Don't know yet. Word is they are going to dig a hole.'

'That is if you haven't dug one for yourself already?' She grins. 'Did you get home to see the wife and kids?'

'Nosey, tonight, aren't you?' he teases, 'I mean, even more than usual?'

Siobhan pouts. 'Just making conversation.'

He makes his way to the other guys on the team at the far end of the pool table. Jimmy is a Glaswegian, East side. He likes to think he is the hard man of the bunch. A man among boys. Nev and he have been heading towards a square up for a few days. His opening gambit is, 'Hae look, the fuckin wanderer returns. Sneaking a day off was yea?'

There are a few jeers from the others, quite happy to see the big quiet man roughed up a bit.

Nev saw it coming. 'Watch your language, pal. Ladies present and all that.'

'Ladies, aye.' Jimmy sneered. 'That where you been all day, is it? Off hame to see your old lady while we all gets the job done? I bet you never telt her about this one though did yea?' Jimmy indicates towards Siobhan. 'Never telt her you was shagging the bar maid after we all went off to bed, eh? Give her one over the pool table, did yea?'

Nev leans down and looks him hard in the eye,

holding his stare. Then he grins. 'At least I can still pull a bird, eh, Jock. Only thing you will have pulled in a long time is right there below yer fat belly, if you can find it.' Nev brushes past him, knocking his shoulder and heading for the toilet. If this Weegie bastard wants to fight, he'll be ready. Jimmy makes a half-hearted attempt to follow but allows the others hold him back.

Siobhan glares at Jimmy from behind the bar.

21st March 2001

In South West Scotland an army Land-rover is driving along a tarmac road through a forest near Johnstonebridge, two soldiers in the front, both wearing berets. They look out at the bleak scenery, snow on the hills in the distance. One says, 'Bloody hell, this is a lively old place. How do folks live out here in the middle of nowhere? I thought the desert was bad enough.'

This is usual soldier banter. The other one takes the bait, keeping up the chat. 'Bunch of sheep-shaggers, I reckon, mate. Wouldn't pull much else at the local disco, eh?' Both men laugh, as the vehicle crosses a cattle grid, rattling the rivets.

Further south, on a farm near Ormskirk in West Lancashire, the team are cleaning up after all the animals have been killed and removed. It's a thankless job, trying to remove germs when you can't see them. As well as the payout for their stock, the farms get a good overhaul, courtesy of the government. Nev is painting a gate while two other guys are sweeping a concrete yard. Danny is a Geordie, one of the quieter lads amongst them. He is aware Nev is a bit more savvy than the rest of them and comes over to speak to him. 'So, we still got a job next week, Nev? You heard anything?'

Nev carries on painting. 'Don't know mate.

Probably. I might not be with you though. Looking for something a bit nearer home. Need to be back near my sheep.'

'You got a farm of your own then?'

'Aye. Just a smallholding, with a few pedigree yows. Good ones, mind. Nae rubbish. Sunk everything I have into them. Took a bit of a risk, really. Like a rush of blood, you nah?'

Danny looks sincere. 'Worried about this disease getting to you?'

'Nah. Should be fine.' Nev is quite confident. 'Well out the way, we are. Miles from owt.'

'Who's looking after them for you?'

'Just the missus. She can cope alright. Her old man is a top sheep farmer. Some of it's rubbed off on her.'

Danny fidgets and looks down at his boots. 'You're not really shagging Siobhan, are you? Playing away, like?'

'Don't you bloody start.' Nev smiles. 'Nah. I got the best wife in the land. Wouldn't swap her for a houseful of that one. We were just talking, that's all. Sometimes nice to unburden yoursel to a stranger.'

The military headquarters that the Brigadier had advised the government was required had been set up in a small village hall called Kelhead, near Annan in Dumfriesshire. Although North of the border in Scotland it is handy for the main road network, as well as being in the thick of the latest round of outbreaks of the disease which had centred itself around Dumfries and Castle Douglas. Captain Moorhouse had been a desk bound officer for most of his career in the forces and had been singled out for this job by the Brigadier himself. Along with Sergeant Dart, the two of them had every holding in a 100-mile radius mapped out and marked, each with its own file on how much livestock it carried, as well as all previous movements. It had taken over a week to sort it all out, with the help of a couple more women cadets, but he was fairly keen that he not only had a handle on the situation now, but had it under strict control. In front of him are a pile of documents and the Captain stamps one with red letters saying CULL, before moving on to the next one. This one is headed 'Newhouse Farm, near Dumfries.' He stands and studies the map on the wall, pinpointing its location. 'Looks this one will have to go. There's no boundary fence between there for miles. Anything could wonder across and rub noses up against the fence. And who knows what's out there on that mountain.'

His Sergeant joins him, checks for a second, and offers his advice. 'Well, you're the boss, Sir, but it looks marginal to me.'

Moorhouse makes his decision and stamps CULL across the document, before moving to the next.

At Newhouse Farm, Helen and Pam are herding seven ewes across the farmyard towards the building. Pam hasn't much idea but is trying. 'Go on you stupid creature. Bloody things ave less brains that my ex-husband!'

Helen is concentrating, aware of their condition. 'Just let them take their time, Pam, don't rush them. They are more pregnant than me!'

An Army Land-rover is coming down the farm track towards them. It stops and a soldier gets out and washes his feet in the trough full of disinfectant before walking towards the gate, holding an envelope. 'Mrs. Lambert?'

Helen looks surprised. 'Yes, that's me.'

'I am afraid I have some bad news for you, about your sheep.' He hands her a letter, and she opens it, and then pulls a hand to her mouth in shock.

Pam looks over her shoulder. 'What is it?'

Helen looks blankly from the sheep, to Pam, and then to the letter. She speaks to the soldier. 'I thought we were safe. Out here, miles from anywhere. How can you do this? How can you do this to our livelihood. What will my husband say?'

'Sorry Ma'am, just following orders.'

She can't control her anger. 'Orders? Whose orders?'

In Lancashire Nev stops painting, realises his phone is vibrating in his pocket. He checks it to see three missed calls, all from Helen. Laying down the brush, he pulls out a cigarette and lights it before dialling the number. 'Hi Love. What's up?'

He listens for a second and then ends the call, angrily throwing his phone at the wall, which smashes.

27th March 2001

Brigadier Hardcastle is silhouetted against a grey Cumbrian sky, surveying the vast area of land around Great Orton Airfield, as Major Richardson approaches. Behind him, a huge green bulldozer is being unloaded off a lorry, it's buzzer blaring to warn everyone that it is reversing blindly. He studies it and then turns to a map in his hand. The Major is a smaller man of similar age, a line of coloured beading decorating his jacket denoting combat.

'You sure you're ready for this, Guy?' The Brigadier speaks with authority but also as a friend.

Guy Richardson glances up towards a cluster of houses away to the left of them. 'Don't think we will be too popular in the village, Sir, but I guess the locals will forgive us if we get it right.'

'I'm sure a few flag-waving housewives won't be enough to stop the operation.' He looks back towards where the machine had already started work. 'How long before we can ship in the first load?'

Guy was quick with an answer, having made and double checked their plans. 'Two days, max. Once we get the first trench dug, we can backfill with lime and then cover as we go. Take a few thousand in on the first day and then we can scale up from there.'

'You'll need to. Logistics are suggesting 20,000 per day. Can you handle that?'

If the enormity of the figure took Guy by surprise, he didn't let it show. 'We can if they can, Sir. That's a lot of lorries but we will set up a one-way road system, in and out. Every truck disinfected before it hits the main road again.'

The ground grumbles as the machine opens up its massive V12 diesel engines, black smoke billowing from two exhaust stacks on the bonnet. Beyond it, two vast low-loader lorries arrive, each with a similar machine on board. A further three are on their way.

'The pits will be four metres deep, and about 150 long. Room for at least 20 of them on the airfield. Reckon the lot will take half a million carcasses.' Guy checks the clip-board he is holding. 'As long as they keep bringing them in, we just keep digging. No point in getting too far in front of ourselves, as the hole will only fill with rainwater.'

Hardcastle has to raise his voice to be heard above the machine. 'Carlisle are still recruiting staff. Got 60 on board yesterday, plus our regulars. Experienced men, most of them. A few ex-soldiers amongst them. You need more drivers here?' He points to the diggers.

The Major shakes his head. 'Got enough regulars on the big machines, working relays around the clock. But we could do with an overspill of truck drivers, so we can keep the supply coming in. And we will need more diggers out there on the farms to load up.'

'OK, I'll see what I can do.' The Brigadier wrings his hands. 'Should be able to bring in some local firms but they will need vetting first. No more cowboys on this operation if we want to get it over and done with.'

In the kitchen at Newhouse Farm, Nev has read the letter from MAFF a dozen times, each time hoping it would say something different. Eventually he screws it up and throws it down on the table.

'I just don't believe it.' He says for the fourth time.

'I know love. It is so unfair.' She wants to cry tears for him. 'Especially out here. But we will get paid out.'

It was probably the wrong thing to say, judging by Nev's reaction. 'I don't want pay. These are my sheep. My choices. My investment. Our investment.' He accepts her hug. 'Our future!'

At the farm gate, a slim man in grey jacket and slacks steps out from his car, takes a briefcase from the boot and pulls on wellington boots. After washing them in the bucket provided, he walks down the drive and is met at the front door by Pam who has watched him arrive through the window.

'David Dickenson,' the man introduces himself. 'Hitherman and Hayes auctioneers. Would you be Mrs. Lambert?'

'Senior!' says Pam. 'Come on in. Neville is in the kitchen.'

David steps inside and greets Nev with a look of greyness. 'Neville. It's been a while. Sorry we can't meet in under happier circumstances.'

'Aye, David. So am I?' Nev shakes his cold hand. 'Take a seat.'

'A cup of tea, Mr. Dickenson?' Helen has met the man before but suspects he won't recall her.

'Coffee, if you have it. One sugar.' He sits and pulls some papers from his briefcase. Then turns to the younger man. 'Just need to complete a few forms, Nev. Then we'll take a look at them.'

'You know, David.' Nev can barely bear to look at the man. A man he knows and has worked with many times. Often shared a pint and a joke. And here he was now, on the side of the executioner. 'I thought we would be safe here. Especially once they got the military in. Seeing all those poor bastards losing their stock. I was almost smug, out here in the wilds.'

'I must admit, I am as surprised as you are.' He shook his head. 'A marginal case, if ever I saw one.'

'Is there a system? Anyone I can appeal to, like?' He faces the man for the first time, hopefully. 'If you say they are healthy, an all.'

Dickenson wasn't going to get drawn in. 'It's not my job to say whether they are healthy or not. I am just here to value them, Neville, that's all. Let's get a price on their head and then see, shall we.'

Originating in Belgium, the Beltex breed of sheep was a hybrid of the Dutch Texel breed, which had been genetically improved by selection of animals with extreme muscling. Imported into the UK by a butcher named Tom Ashton in the early 1990s, the same man responsible for bringing over the Belgian Blue cattle breed, the name Beltex had stuck. Over the next decade a number of forward-thinking breeders from England, Scotland and Ireland imported the best Belgium females they could find as demand for this meaty carcassed animal grew exponentially. By the turn of the century butchers were clamouring to get lambs from this breed which offered superior carcasses and a better return. The eight ewes that Nev now owned were from some of the best bloodlines in the breed, something which had reflected in their cost. David and Nev stood at the gate to the barn, admiringly.

'They're looking well, Nev. How far off lambing?'

'Just days now. Already had a pair a few days ago. Over there.' He points at the ewe with two young lambs in a pen on their own, the lambs sucking.

'That's a braw Beltex tup lamb, Neville. It's a braw flock of Beltex in fact.' He pulls back his cap and runs his hands through his hair. 'Dam this bloody disease.' He climbs the railing to take a closer look. 'Don't mind if I..?'

'Be my guest.'

David scans the pen and then looks back to the lamb. 'A few thou, at least!

'What for the lot o them?' Nev throws up his hands. 'Jesus fuck!'

'No, just for that one, Nev. That lamb. Could easy make a couple of grand. Well bred. Plenty of arse. Good skin. Aye, could well be a champion in the making.'

Nev's whole demeanour changes as he takes this in. Eventually he says slowly. 'You saying a four-day old lamb is worth a couple of grand?'

'Not saying it is, but that's not to say it wouldn't be, one day.'

The two men look at each other for a second and then back to the sheep.

It's Nev's turn to break the silence. 'Are you saying you can value animals on their potential rather than what they are worth now?'

'Well, I couldn't with the other ones. I know what you paid for them, as I sold them to you, and that is pretty much all they are worth at this point in time. But with lambs at foot? Well, each lamb has a value.'

'Bloody hell.' Nev's voice goes up an octave. 'Let me get this straight? If I get lambs out of these ewes, you will double their valuations?'

'Treble, I would say.'

The bleat of a ewe breaks the silence, as the bizarreness of the situation hits home. 'And then they all have to be killed?'

David just nods.

'So I bring them into the world, David? Take your money. And then you kill them?'

'Not my money, Nev. It's the government's money. When is the slaughter scheduled for?'

'Monday or Tuesday.'

David looks around, as though checking he wouldn't be overheard. 'Let's see, today is Thursday. You want me to postpone this for a couple of days...maybe have some more lambs by then, over the weekend. That one looks like she could produce tonight.'

'No, I bloody well don't. That's immoral, and cruel. And. And bloody ridiculous!' The shout Nev reacts with makes David take a step back.

'Just offering.' He manages, 'It might be immoral,

but it is perfectly legal.'

But Nev hasn't finished shouting. 'Legal? Legal? How can any of this be bloody legal. Killing innocent healthy animals?'

Already writing on a form, David touches him on the shoulder. 'Tell you what I will do, lad. I will complete this form, with the values on it. 800 pounds each for the ewes. 300 for that ewe lamb, and 1500 for the ram lamb. I won't put a date on it for now, but you can fill that in yourself. If more lambs are born before the slaughter boys arrive, give me a call and we can re-look at it. OK?'

30th March 2001

The rain is just starting to fall as Nev turns his pick-up off the main road and down through a village of cosy houses. A yellow sign indicates 'Airfield entrance' and he slows and follows it. As he reaches the centre of the small community a number of people line the sides of the roads waving home-made banners. One says, 'STOP THE KILLING FIELDS' while another is emblazoned 'KEEP YOUR DEATHS OUT OF OUR VILLAGE! He pulls his pick-up into a car-park and pushes through the protesters heading towards a portakabin. In the distance he counts at least 20 bulldozers at work, pushing soil around like kids' toys on a beach. As he reaches the end of the line of unhappy locals, a voice calls to him that he recognises.

It is Ross Davidson. 'You working here now then, Neville?'

Nev stands squarely in front of the smaller man. 'You can get fucked, and all!'

'I saw your name was on the list. For the cull.' Ross is wary. 'Want to talk about it?'

'I should be punching you in the face. Bastard, writing all that bollocks about me.'

The journalist goes on the defensive. 'I know you won't believe me, but it wasn't me that added all that stuff about your military career. I sold the story to the

Daily Mail and next thing they had added a load of stuff I didn't even know about it. If you want my theory...'

It's been a long few days, few weeks, and Nev's temper is frayed to breaking point. He grabs Ross by the neck, pushing him backwards. 'Aye, theory, that's all you fuckers have got, isn't it. And what you don't know, you make up. Should have never spoken to you in the first place, you wanker!'

The man just about shakes himself free. 'You don't have to believe me, but the government spin doctors got to that piece, via Rupert Murdoch.'

'That bastard?'

'Yes, that bastard. Look, I might be able to help you set the record straight.'

'Aye, and print more lies.' Nev stares at him with bloodshot eyes. 'What's in it for me this time?'

'I saw the cull list, and there are a number of culling cases marked 'marginal'. He takes a breath. 'Your farm was one of them.'

'So?'

'So, if we shout loud enough, maybe they will over-turn it. You know? State your case, then use the story that you were the one who protested that the government bring in the army, and the first thing they did was shoot your sheep.'

'Except they haven't shot them, mate. Just making me suffer a little bit longer.'

'Exactly!' Ross admits. 'We don't have much time.'

Nev still isn't buying it. 'I dunno, pal. I think I have

done enough public pleading for now, don't you? Hasn't done me much good, so far?'

With that Nev walks on past a line of ticker tape, which is patrolled by a soldier. He shows a paper to the guard and heads towards the cabin.

'Think about it, Neville.' Ross shouts behind him. 'Even if it just bought you a few more days? You got my number.'

As Nev enters the cabin, the Brigadier is coming out. The two men stop and look at each other for a second. 'Excuse me,' mutters the officer.

Nev whips up a smart salute. 'Private Lambert, reporting for civilian duty, Sir!'

Hardcastle is about to walk on but stops. 'Lambert, did you say?'

'Yes, Sir.' Nev's voice took on a clipped note. 'Served with the LI, in Iraq, Sir. Sniper, Sir. Under your command.'

The officer looked at him for the first time. 'Sniper, eh? Well, you'll certainly come in handy around here then, Mr. Lambert. Good to have you on board.'

Nev salutes again. 'Sir!' This time the officer salutes back.

As Nev goes inside the portakabin the Brigadier heads over towards a large pit that has been dug. He watches a lorry arrive alongside and reverse towards the hole. As the back raises on hydraulics, the tail gate opens and 100 rotting decaying sheep slide out and down the four metres to the bottom, making a thudding sound. The Brigadier, along with Guy

Richardson, is standing 20 feet away and he pulls a handkerchief to his mouth. 'Bloody hell!'

'That was a nasty one.' Guy chips in. 'Some of these carcasses have been sitting around for over a week.'

The senior officer turns away from the smell and noise so he can speak. 'How's it going?'

'All under control, Sir, although I hadn't quite realised how much of a back log there was. Will take a few days to clear it. Have we started shooting yet?'

'Due to start today.'

Guy nods understandingly. 'Would be better if they hang on another day or two if possible?' he suggests. 'Might ease up this stench a bit. Natives are getting restless. Not a good time to be hanging out their washing!'

'I will see what I can do.' The Brig replies. 'The number of cases is slowing but still some more urgent than others. How's morale in the ranks?'

Guy shouts above the noise of another machine pushing the carcasses along in the pit below them. 'A few screwed-up noses but these are trained men, Sir. They don't stop to think about it. Don't get time to think about it. Just getting on with their jobs.'

'And the new recruits?'

'Most of them seem OK, Sir. We have put the more squeamish ones on the lorry cleaning. And a there are few HGV drivers among them. Still a few new ones arriving.'

'So I see.' The Brigadier moves closer to Richardson's ear. 'I met one just now, think I have encountered him before. Served under me in the desert. A sniper. Bit of a trouble-maker, if I recall. Got caught up behind enemy lines by Saddam's boys. Took a good hiding and then threatened to shoot his mouth off about our tactics if we didn't let him go. Name of Lambert. Keep your eye on that one, Major.'

Nev has signed the relevant paperwork and had been issued with a security pass that allowed him access in and out of the site, as well as keys to a Scania. Considering his most recent credentials as a lorry driver it was a fairly obvious decision to put him on trucks carrying the carcasses from the surrounding area to Great Orton. He has just made his first pick-up and arrives back in the lane near the site. With this number of vehicles arriving in such a rural spot it was inevitable that there would be a queue both in and out of the place. He eyes the one in front, its tarpaulin barely hiding the mass of dead sheep underneath it. To both sides of the lorries are small cottages with neat lawns, one with a tree-house built into an old apple tree. A woman mouths something to him from outside so he flips down the window, just to hear her point of view. 'You lot should be ashamed. Bringing all those dead animals through here. Disrupting the peace. Spreading your nasty germs. And that honk, stinking out the whole district.'

He just nods expressionlessly to her, before putting the window back up and reaching for his mobile phone. When he dials Helen, she answers on the third ring. 'Any news?' he asks.

'Still nothing from the military yet. But I think one of the ewes might be lambing. She is restless, standing up and then digging up the straw. Should I put her in a pen on her own, do you think?'

These are difficult words for any shepherd to hear under these circumstances. 'Do your best for her love. I know it's hard. Tough to think the lambs won't even see the grass, but gotta do what we can, make sure she's OK and not suffering.'

'I'll try and get them alive,' she says, hopefully.

'Aye, do that pet. And not just because of the money. Do what you can, for her sake.' He lights a cigarette and puts the window down a touch. The woman is still shouting her protests outside, but he ignores her and continues. 'Helen. You want to give me the number for the ministry? I'll try and call them, see if there is an appeal procedure. You never know, worth a try.'

Helen looks it up off a headed document on the table and reads it out while Nev scribbles it down. The lorry in front moves on, so he ends the conversation. 'Thanks Love. Gotta go. I'll be home tonight.'

It was a long day and quite boring once you got over the extent of the operation and the smell of rotting animals. The shifts would be long, but the pay was by the hour and Nev would pull in more money on this work than his regular job with Armstrongs. And it meant he could get home every night.

It was gone eight when his wife put down his dinner and sat opposite him. The day had ended slightly better. 'Great job. That's a decent ewe lamb there. Must have been a bit of a squeeze getting it out? You did well.'

Helen accepts the praise. In reality it had been a difficult job, getting Pam to help her as well as she pulled the lamb out by the front legs using all her strength, and a couple of pieces of string. She hoped her next childbirth would be easier, but she let it go at that. 'Well, they both seem healthy, that's the main thing. Did you get through to MAFF?'

'I managed to get past the switchboard but got stonewalled after that.' Nev tucked into a slice of gammon. 'MAFF can pass the buck now, can't they? *The culling decision is no longer ours*', that's what they said. It was in the hands of the Ministry of Defence. As if I am going to call them up, eh?'

His mother takes exception to that. 'Why not? You worked for them. Went to war for them. Surely they owe you a favour or two?'

'I am not sure it works like that, Pam,' Helen tells her.

'Aye.' Nev nods. 'And anyway, that was then, and this is now. Did I mention that my old CO was running the show down there in Wigton? Bumped into him this morning, although I don't think he recognised me. Those guys see a lot of soldiers, but I sometimes wonder if they actually see any of them at all, as anything other than cannon fodder. He's a man who gets what he wants, and no mistake. A real decision maker.'

Helen gets up and puts the kettle on, her back to the table.

'That reporter was there as well,' Nev adds. 'The one who got me in the papers.'

'What, Ross whatshisname? I bet he steered well clear of you?'

'Strangely enough, no. Came straight up to me, bold as brass. Trying to offer me a deal.'

Pam stands up from the table as well. 'Come on you two, time for Coronation Street. George is quite a fan, aren't you, George?'

'Yes, Granny,' says the boy.

As they leave the room Helen asks, 'What sort of a deal?'

'Ah, you na how they are, those hacks. Just wants some more tears on the page. Said he had checked the list and seen my name on it.'

'What list?'

'The list of farms designated to cull. Said ours was marginal.' He sniffs. 'I could have told him that, stuck out here, miles from anywhere.'

'So, what was he offering?' She pours boiling water into three cups.

'Oh, says that I should stand up and start spouting again. Along the lines of 'I did my stint in the army, and it was me who called in the army to this job and now this is how they repay me, by taking out our flock'.'

She spun round. 'Do you think it would work?'

'Not a chance.' Nev shakes his head, reaching for a cigarette now the kids have gone. 'The army don't read the papers, love. It would just wind people up. Probably lose my job in the process.'

'But if enough people heard about it. Peer pressure and all that?'

'Nah. It won't work.' He lights one up. 'Marginal or

not, the bullets will be here soon enough.'

'What happened to the man who never gives up, Nev? That was you - just a short while ago?'

Nev just sighs. 'I think the whole thing is getting me down, Helen. Getting us all down. Let's just get it over with and get on with our lives. Keeping pedigree sheep was crazy idea anyway. For a chav bastard like me. Just take the money and run.'

'Aw, come on.' She puts an arm around him. 'Never let them grind you down. That's what you used to say.'

'You saying I should call him? Drag us all through it again?'

'Could he get you back on TV?'

'I doubt it.' He gives her a peck on the cheek. 'Story isn't so hot now. Viewers getting bored of farmers crying crocodile tears and then heading off with the loot. You should have seen the locals near that burial site. Thought they were going to take pot shots at us.'

'You make us sound like the bad guys?'

'Good and bad in everyone? That's what they say. Yin and yang.'

'You with your bloody yin and yang theories.' She punches him lightly on the shoulder. Then she chucks him the phone and Ross's card. 'Yin and yang. Those who try, and those who don't. Which one are you?'

1st April 2001

The two men sit opposite each other, Nev cautious and on guard, Ross aware he is not flavour of the month. It is 9.30am and they are in a small cafe just outside Wigton, which serves all-day breakfast with as much grease as you could eat.

'You owe me, pal.' Nev glares at his adversary, holding his eyes as he speaks. 'And if anything gets printed about me that I haven't told you, I'll be gunning for you, and no mistake.'

'Aye, so you said on the phone.'

'Well, make sure you remember it.' Nev reminds him. 'You owe me!'

Ross is getting tired of the threats now. He had hoped that the man would understand that the piece had been tampered with by an editor under orders. 'Look, you want to keep your sheep. I want to at least make amends. Let's just stick to the facts here.'

'Facts. That's rich, coming from you.'

Ross does his best to ignore that and pulls out his notebook. 'I have an idea of how we can canvass for an appeal, but I will need more from you.'

'Like what?'

Ross knows his next line will hit a raw nerve. 'You

were posted behind enemy lines, right?'

'How the hell did you know that?' Nev's hackles are rising again.

'Never mind how I know. I just did some digging, OK? Just tell me some more.'

'And have you print it. No way Ho-sey!'

Ross sighs. 'I won't print it. Not this time. Not without your say so. You have my word.'

Back at Foot and Mouth's northern HQ, Captain Moorhouse and his Sergeant believe they have the situation under control. Dart has made tea and sips his from a white tin mug. 'Got a call from MAFF in Page Street this morning. Said they have had quite a few calls about some of these marginal farm culls. Wanting to know if there was an appeal procedure?'

Moorhouse doesn't look up from his map. 'Trying to undermine our decisions, eh?'

'I guess. Certainly making us out to be the bad guys around here.'

'No surprise there, then.' The Captain looks up this time. 'And do we?

'Do we what?'

'Have an appeal procedure?'

Both officers laugh. 'Ref's decision is final!'

Despite being a military man through and through, it would be a poor show if the top brass had to travel around in Land-rovers all the while, with their hard suspension and solid seats. When not being delivered by helicopter, Brigadier Hardcastle chose a more comfortable mode of transport to get him from Scotland to Devon and London, and wherever else this damn disease was likely to pop up next. Reclining into his leather seat in the back of a top range Mercedes was surely one of the perks one should expect for a man in his position. As he reads through a memo, his eyes are closing until his mobile phone sounds. He picks it up. 'Robert Hardcastle!'

'Brigadier, my name is Davidson,' says the caller. 'Daily Mail. Could I have a quick comment from you about the progress of the operation in Cumbria?

'How the hell did you get this number?' The Brig bristles at the thought of his private number being handed out to all and sundry. 'There is a press office for this sort of thing.

'Yes, Sir,' says Ross 'I am aware of that, but I was after a little more information. Your personal comments on the excellent job the men are doing up there.'

Hardcastle settles a bit. 'Well, I can only reiterate what you just said, Mr. Davidson. Our national forces have combined with some local men and Operation Peninsula is all going according to plan.'

Ross keeps the conversation going, knowing he only has a few seconds before the senior officer ends it. 'Can I ask what your take is on culling marginal farms which are not directly affected?'

'Um. That is not really a subject for discussion. The culling decisions are made based on sound evidence, that's all you need to know. Goodbye…'

'Wait!' Davidson jumps in. 'What if I told you that quite a high-profile farm has been selected for culling, despite it being over a mile from its nearest neighbour and has had no stock near its boundary for at least three months.'

'I am not sure I understand. What does this have to do with me?'

'I am doing a story on it, Sir.

'A story? I see.' The Brigadier senses a game when he hears one. 'You are phoning me on a private number to tell me you are doing a random story on one farm that is to be culled. Is there anything else you can tell me? If it is high-profile, then maybe I should know more?'

'What, so that you can call in a few favours at Fleet Street and get it rejected?'

'Look Davidson, I am a busy man.' The red button was being reached for again. 'If you have something to say, then out with it. Or stop pestering me.'

'The farm belongs to one of your own, Sir.' The reporter tries not to sound patronising. 'One of your soldiers. Or at least he was, once.'

'A name, please?' snaps the officer. 'Give me a name?'

'Not until I have your assurance that he will keep his employment, and that you will re-open his case.'

'And why would I do that?' Hardcastle breathes deeply. 'Are you blackmailing me, Davidson?'

'Not at all, Sir.' Ross has been waiting for that word and is ready for it. 'I have a story, I was just after a comment. It's a good story. Well, good from a reader point of view. I am not so sure you would like it. All I am saying is that it doesn't have to be printed, you get me?'

'You are blackmailing me, you little shit!' The line is silent for a few seconds. The Brig sighs. 'What is it that you want?'

'My guy has some top breeding sheep. He is a good guy, an honest man, just starting out. He is on your side, Sir. And, for the record, he knows nothing of this conversation.' That bit was true.

'And what if I believe you?'

Ross is only a fraction away from pleading but tries to keep a forceful tone. 'He just deserves another chance, that's all I am saying. A chance to keep what is his, a chance to keep his dreams alive, Sir. He did some dirty work for you, some time back. I think perhaps, now is your chance to let him off the hook.'

Hardcastle had played hardball enough times to bury this suggestion. 'I'm sorry, but even if this man has a good case, it's not up to me. I don't decide on the cull, it is not up to me to interfere.'

Ross refrains from using the word 'rubbish'. 'Your people all answer to you, Sir. Everyone does, indirectly. I am sure there could be an appeal procedure put in place.'

'Give me his name, I'll see what I can do.'

'Not until I have your word, Sir.' Ross feels the man drop a guard but knows it can come back up at any time. 'Not until you assure me you will put in a good word for him and re-examine his case.'

'In exchange for what?'

'In exchange for some information I have about operation Desert Storm. And about how you posted men in highly dangerous situations, behind the front line.'

'That was all in the past, son.' The Brig has lost sincerity now. 'Nobody cares anymore.'

Ross throws in the strike. 'Then, in the past is perhaps where it needs to stay, Sir? With what's going on, and your senior position, it is probably the last thing you need, making the headlines about some past misdemeanours.'

Ross lets it hang so long, he checks the phone to see if the line is still active.

At last the submission came. 'Alright, hold that story for now. You have my word I will look into it. And you don't need to tell me the name, I think I have that worked out. Lambert, right?'

This time the line does go dead.

Ross's next call won't be much easier, as he scrolls through the contact list and hits the speed dial.

Nev answers. 'Yes, Ross?' Listens. 'You did what!? For fuck's sake, man. That's exactly what I told you not to do. You'll get me fired!' He pulls a cigarette from a near empty pack, still listening to the call. 'Well, you'd better be right about this. Or we are both in the shit!'

2nd April 2001

Sergeant Dart answers the phone after four rings. The shifts have been long, and he is not really in the mood for any conversation, as he utters the words, 'Foot & Mouth HQ.' The sound of the caller straightens him up and his tone changes instantly. 'Oh, hello, Sir. Yes. Yes, he is right here.' Covering the receiver, he says, 'It's the Brigadier, for you, Captain.'

Moorhouse greets his superior wisely. 'Yes, Sir, good afternoon. How can I help?' While listening he raises an eyebrow to his colleague before answering again. 'An appeal procedure? Er, no, Sir. I don't think…' Dart watches him as his face reddens. 'Yes, Sir. I am sure it could be set up.' Moorhouse scribbles down the word 'Appeal' on to a jotter. 'Right now? Yes, Sir, we will get on to it straight away.'

Unlike the top brass, regular soldiers do not get to travel in comfort, as anyone who has taken a ride in a military four-tonner will advocate. For one thing, the cushions in the back are pretty thin and for another, the springs are overly solid, built to withstand some pretty rough terrain. The terrain this one is motoring along is a narrow hillside track and one sergeant, along with two other soldiers are sitting in the back peering out at the high hills on either side. Each has a rifle.

When it comes to comfort, Nev's cab is somewhere in between the squaddies and their master's, as he motors along the A66 towards Stainton, breaking the speed limit. His phone rings and he answers, not recognising the number. 'Yes?'

'Er, Mr. Lambert. This is Major Richardson at Great Orton. I wondered if you could pop in and see me in my office when you arrive with your next load.'

'Yes, Sir. What's it about, only I was hoping to be home early tonight.'

The call is already ended.

A few miles later Nev climbs down from the cab to watch a JCB loading sheep carcasses into the back of his wagon. Blood drips down the sides and on to the wheels. The digger itself is no longer its usual yellow colour, more of a reddy-brown. Nev tries not to retch.

The road the army truck is travelling on has turned into a farm track and all three of its personnel in the rear can feel it, in their rears. The driver is glad he is the driver.

In a small office somewhere in England, Ross Davidson is typing an email in to his laptop. The subject line reads 'Operation Desert Storm'. The recipient is Brigadier Robert Hardcastle.

An hour later Nev joins the queue of lorries in Great Orton village which is shorter than last time. Slowly, he edges forwards until he eventually gets through the gate into the site, stopping to speak to a guard through the window. 'Sheep, this time. Same place?'

'Yes, same as the others,' says the man. 'Should have that plot filled by tonight so they can close it in. On you go.'

As Nev swings round into the site, he sees that another hole has been opened up beyond the one currently in use. Sheep and cattle carcasses mingle together twenty or thirty deep, sinking as more are piling in. By tomorrow they will be covered over, buried in their own mass grave. A large metal-wheeled digger carries a bucket full of lime down into the hole, driving over some of the bodies which pop under its weigh. The lime will soon degrade the flesh to nothing, but the animals will never quite disappear. Nev pulls the wagon to one side, climbs down and heads towards the large block of portakabins and goes to a reception hatch. 'Here to see Major Richardson. Neville Lambert.'

A receptionist picks up a phone and dials. 'Could you let the Major know Mr. Lambert is here to see him, please? Thanks.' She turns back to Nev. 'Up the stairs, second on the right.'

The four-tonner slows to a halt and the soldiers are glad of the respite, while the driver climbs from the cab and dials a number on his mobile phone. 'Hello, Mrs Lambert…' The call ends itself and he curses. 'No bloody reception in this valley. Bet they still have outside toilets!' He reaches back into the cab and blows the horn. Then reading from a document on a clip-board he goes around the back of the lorry. 'Come on lads, this one won't take long. Only a few of them.'

The three soldiers jump down, rifles in hand.

Down in the farmyard, Pam is holding the head of a ewe while Helen pulls a pair of back legs, straining. 'Bloody thing. I hope mine comes out easier than this?' she mutters.

They both hear the horn blowing. It is Pam who acknowledges the noise. 'That'll be the executioners then?'

Without warning the lamb comes out with a pop and Helen nearly goes over backwards. She holds it up by its back legs and swings it, a manoeuvre well known to shepherds throughout the globe. It takes its first breath. It is alive. For now.

'Go and stall them, will you please, Pam. At least until this thing gets a suck of milk. Give them a cup of tea or something, eh. Use your charm.'

'Charm some young men?' Pam grins. 'At last I get a decent job around here!'

For the size of the small makeshift office, the layout is impressive, with maps on each wall almost making it like a 3-D movie. Major Richardson is fairly unmistakable. A blueprint of all the Majors Nev has met and taken orders from in the past. He stands up. 'Neville, is it? Take a seat.'

Nev sits. Like a schoolboy summoned to the Headmaster's office with no idea why. 'Sir.'

'I gather you were one of us, once?' the Major says, pretending to read it from a resume. 'Did some service?'

'I did my time, yes.'

Guy checks down the document he has read once

already. 'Medical discharge, wasn't it?'

'Sort of.' Nev is confused as to why he is wasting his time here when both men have better things to be doing.

'And you were paid off?'

'I got some money when I left, yes. Could I ask what this is about, Sir? Only I have some pressing business back home to attend to.'

'It won't take long, Neville,' the Major says calmly. 'Just want to clear up a couple of things.'

'About my army career? That was long ago, dead and buried, Sir. I don't really want to talk about it.'

Guys looks up at him. 'You did give statements though. Didn't you? Were even offered promotion to Sergeant? But you preferred to question our methods of action.'

The penny starts to drop. 'That was back then, Sir. I did what I was told to do, but...'

'You were behind the line, weren't you? Went a bit too far forward?'

Nev eyeballs the officer. He is not serving any more. No charge for insubordination for a civilian. 'I did what I thought was right.'

Richardson wasn't reading now. Just returning the ex-soldier's stare. 'But you over-stepped the mark, didn't you? Your remit was to stay on our side of the line, and pick off designated targets?'

Nev says nothing, always the best policy under interrogation.

'But you got a bit too cock sure of yourself, didn't you?' The Major fires off his accusation. 'Decided to move forward on your own initiative - without authorisation?'

'I was fighting a war, Sir.'

'We were all fighting a bloody war, Private. But fighting a war is about team work. You went out on your own, didn't you? Took the law in to your own hands. Went on a bloodthirsty killing spree. And then got caught, didn't you? Nearly gave the whole damn game away.'

Silence again. Somewhere a clock is ticking, much slower than Nev's pulse.

'Didn't you, Neville?' the officer repeats quietly.

Suspecting his job is on the line, Nev chooses to speak up at last. 'I was authorised, Sir.'

'You were sent?' Guy doesn't believe him. 'By whom?'

'I'd rather not say, Sir.'

Guy looks back to the paperwork a while longer. 'You'd rather not say? Is that you keeping silent on military matters? Or you making up lies?'

Nev has no more to lose now. Just wants this over with. 'I know when to keep my mouth shut, Sir. I did then. And I do now.'

'Are you sure?' Here comes the crunch, and the Major is about to unload it. 'I am reliably informed that you, for the second time, suggest your silence has a price. You got away with that, once.' He stands up. 'It won't happen twice. Not surprisingly, the army isn't very keen on blackmail.'

Nev stands too and makes to leave. 'Sir, if you don't mind, I need to get home to my sheep.'

At Newhouse Farm, two soldiers are standing at the kitchen door, while the other one watches Helen carrying a live lamb into a pen, its mother following.

'You really don't need to do that, madam.' His voice is English, Birmingham perhaps.

'Yes, I bloody well do.' Her teeth are gritted. 'It's the least she deserves.'

Pam takes centre stage. 'Come on in officers. Let me get you a nice cuppa. Come in, out of the cold.'

The sergeant, who is the nearest to an officer among them, holds up his hand. 'Sorry, Ma'am. But we are on a strict time schedule this afternoon. Just need this paperwork signed off and we will go about our business.'

Before Nev can reach the door, Major Richardson hands him a document, one he has been holding in his hand. 'Ah, yes.' He says. 'A matter of your sheep. Newhouse Farm, isn't it? Nice remote little place, out in the wilds, where you can keep yourself to yourself, eh? Didn't we pay for that?

The man's tone is patronising which rankles with Nev. 'It's a working farm, Sir. Or at least it was, until today.' He takes the document and looks at it. The word APPEAL is printed at the top. 'What's this?'

'I suggest you fill it in and sign it pretty damn quick.'

Nev fights back an uncontrollable tear. 'It's too late, the deed has been done.' He heads for the door again.

'Not necessarily.' The officer has hardened. 'One phone call from me and it's surprising how things can change.' He hands Nev a second piece of paper, this one headed 'Official Secrets Act.'

At Newhouse Farm, Helen stands with her head in her hands. Beside her, two soldiers line up a sheep each in their sights. She wants to shout at them, scream even. Inside she feels her baby kick for the first time. She is so glad Nev isn't here, although she wants to hug him tightly. Somewhere in the distance a phone rings. Then there is some shouting from a figure running through the farmyard. It's Pam. 'Which one is Sergeant Lewis? A phone call for you. Say's it's from HQ. Says it's urgent!'

Inside his portakabin stronghold, Major Richardson gives an order. 'Oh, and you had better sign this one too, Private Lambert. It basically says you will maintain your silence on this matter, indefinitely.'

It's dark now in the farmyard, although the light is on in the barn. A ewe is lying on her side, covered in blood. There is more blood on the straw around her, as well as on the stone wall.

A lamb gives a single bleat.

The ewe opens one eye when she hears it.

A man in rubber gloves is packing up his medical kit.

'No wonder she needed a caesarean, I think that must be the biggest lamb I have delivered this year!'

Nev holds the new-born lamb up to head height. 'Aye, and hopefully one of the best and ah.'

In an office in England, Ross checks down an email he has written, and the presses the delete button. He speaks to himself. 'Not everyone needs to know everything, eh?'

THE END

Epilogue

From 24th March to 30th September 2001, 460,000 carcasses were buried at Great Orton Airfield during Operation Peninsula.

At its height, more than 10,000 vets, soldiers, field staff and contractors were engaged in fighting the Foot and Mouth disease outbreak.

In mid-April 2001, up to 100,000 animals per day were being killed.

In total, nearly six million animals were slaughtered, either as a direct result of the disease, or on welfare grounds.

The cost to the tax payer was approximately three billion pounds.

The estimated cost to the private sector through loss of revenue was around a further five billion.

The initial outbreak of the disease was

suspected to be caused by meat illegally imported in a suitcase from the Far East.

Tony Blair and the Labour Government got re-elected in June 2001 by a large majority for a further four-year term, in one of the lowest turnouts at the polls the country had seen in recent years.

Author's note

Having been a farmer all my life, along with my father I was involved in a number of pedigree breeds of sheep over four decades. The entrepreneur that he was, my father, together with my brother, specialised in the Beltex breed whereas I built up a flock of Texels. Both were quite successful.

In 2000 we purchased a Beltex ram for a considerable amount, in a share with a breeder in Wigton, Cumbria. The outbreak of Foot and Mouth put paid to him and he now lies buried in a large hole at Great Orton.

At the same time, a case half a mile from our farm in Worcestershire saw us closed down, right in the middle of lambing. The government moved in and shot all the animals on that place and then left them to rot for three days, with the wind blowing our way. I can still hear those bullets and smell that odour. Then they burned them all, the smoke coming not only into our sheep-shed but the farmhouse too. With my flock starting to hit the success trail, I believe that year I bred my best lambs ever. For days we sat and awaited our fate. Through a contact, I got a slot on prime-time TV via a webcam from the farmhouse. What I said during those interviews is reflected in this story.

As with this story, our flocks did survive the cull, but movement restrictions shut the whole place down making it impossible to sell stock for over a year. A lot of my friends weren't quite so lucky, as the outbreak took out some of the best genetics in the UK. The following year, with the restrictions lifted, I won the ewe lamb class at the Royal Show, but my heart had gone out of the job. Another few cases two years later revived the restrictions again and I sold the flock soon afterwards.

I promised my father that one day I would write a story about those torrid times, and that is where this came from.

Originally written as a screenplay, I attempted to sell it to the BBC and other production companies, but to no avail. Maybe it would be a bit too emotional for prime-time TV. Now, in January 2020, the farming industry is taking such a battering from the growing ignorance of the vegan sector that it spurred me to retrieve this screen-drama from my archives and re-write it as a novel. Hence it is written in the present tense and very dialogue driven, not the conventional way to write a story I agree.

I would suspect it has brought back some memories, not necessarily good ones, to many a reader. It certainly left me emotionally drained when I wrote it.

There are still many stories that I have heard about this subject that have not been revealed here, the ones which may forever remain untold.

Thank you for reading this, my 40th book.

Kind regards

Andy Frazier

January 2020

For information on this book, any other books by this author, or the screenplays available, please contact

Andy Frazier

www.andyfrazier

andyfrazier@hotmail.co.uk